The Politics of Cancer

The Politics of Cancer

Malignant Indifference

Wendy N. Whitman Cobb

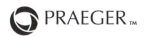

PRAEGER™

An Imprint of ABC-CLIO, LLC

Santa Barbara, California • Denver, Colorado

Library of Congress Cataloging-in-Publication Data

Names: Cobb, Wendy N. Whitman, author.
Title: The politics of cancer : malignant indifference / Wendy N. Whitman Cobb.
Description: Santa Barbara, California : Praeger, an Imprint of ABC-CLIO, LLC,
    [2017] | Includes bibliographical references and index.
Identifiers: LCCN 2016052460 (print) | LCCN 2017001454 (ebook) |
    ISBN 9781440853302 (hard copy : alk. paper) | ISBN 9781440853319 (ebook)
Subjects: LCSH: Cancer—Government policy—United States. | Cancer—Law and
    legislation—United States. | Health policy—United States.
Classification: LCC RC276 .C63 2017 (print) | LCC RC276 (ebook) |
    DDC 362.19699/4—dc23
LC record available at https://lccn.loc.gov/2016052460

ISBN: 978-1-4408-5330-2
EISBN: 978-1-4408-5331-9

21 20 19 18 17   1 2 3 4 5

This book is also available as an eBook.

Praeger
An Imprint of ABC-CLIO, LLC

ABC-CLIO, LLC
130 Cremona Drive, P.O. Box 1911
Santa Barbara, California 93116-1911
www.abc-clio.com

This book is printed on acid-free paper ∞

Manufactured in the United States of America

For Dad

Contents

Preface

I remember the phone call, or rather, the phone calls. I was an undergraduate in college. My phone had been on silent for the night, and I woke up to half a dozen missed calls. My dad had gone to the hospital in the middle of the night and would soon be having his gallbladder taken out due to an incidence of gall stones. In what would be a stroke of luck, the gallbladder attack led to the discovery of a mass on my dad's kidney. Cancer. A word that no one in my family said and purposefully avoided. A lifetime smoker, we all knew that eventually the years of smoking would lead to this, but we didn't anticipate it so soon.

Kidney cancer is incredibly hard to detect until it's too late. By the time it becomes symptomatic, it has most likely metastasized to other locations throughout the body. At that point, it becomes practically incurable. Catching my dad's cancer early allowed surgeons to remove the kidney along with the cancer, supposedly curing it. Within the span of a month, my dad had been through two major surgeries and had the surgical scars across his stomach to prove it.

Once the kidney and the cancer had been removed, we were assured by the surgeon that no further treatment was needed. My dad would have full-body scans about twice a year for five years with no recurrences. The memories faded along with the scars, and my dad continued to smoke. Of course we would all tell him he needed to quit, but as it usually is with such a strong addiction, it would prove difficult for Dad to break the habit. When he would see his primary care doctor, he would proclaim Dad to be the healthiest smoker he had ever seen. That is until six years after the original occurrence.

Dad would discover the cancer had returned in another "lucky" illness. He was struck with a bad cold and the coughing had become severe. The doctor ordered chest x-rays and along with a case of pneumonia, noted five masses near or on his lungs. Not wanting to worry us kids needlessly, Mom and Dad kept the findings to themselves for the time being while waiting for more tests and an appointment with an oncologist. My grandmother had been told, and she was the one who gave me the heads up that something was on my dad's lungs. Since I was little, I always needed to know things in advance and so it didn't strike me out of the blue when Mom and Dad did finally call and tell me that the doctors suspected lung cancer.

Thus began our family education in cancer. This time, we had to say the word. We had to confront it. Given my dad's history of smoking, lung cancer is what we all had expected would eventually affect him. However, we were told that without a biopsy, the doctors couldn't say for sure what *kind* of cancer it is; it could be lung or it could be the kidney cancer that had metastasized. It didn't matter the location as much as the type of cells that had begun to grow out of control. Further testing would indeed show that the five masses on Dad's lungs and adrenal glands were the kidney cancer come back with a vengeance. Although we will never be sure whether it was the smoking that caused it or his bad habit of working extremely hard and many times on the night shift, there has been a demonstrated link between smoking and many other types of cancers, including kidney.

I didn't break down until I got the call that yes, this was kidney cancer and, worse yet, it was stage IV and inoperable. Something about not being able to do anything about it surgically was what affected me so deeply. We are brought up believing that these types of things could simply be cut out of the body and expunged in a highly surgical manner. However, cutting open a chest and digging into glands and organs, although removing the masses, does not guarantee the elimination of cancerous cells that have already spread throughout the body. And cutting into those masses could only propagate the cancer further. The only hope was toxic chemotherapy with the aim of shrinking the tumors.

By this time, I had received a PhD and was teaching in Oklahoma, hundreds of miles away from my family in Florida. My husband, an officer in the Army, was not with me at the time either. It was myself and my dog alone with fears of losing my dad within a relatively short period of time. I flew home over my spring break, which was about a month after the diagnosis. Dad and I went to a spring training baseball game together, a sport that we had shared since I was little and he was my Little League coach. I held back the tears as I tried to take in every memory of that game, which could be my last one with my dad. Although he doesn't share his emotions and feelings that often, I have to believe he was also thinking the same thing.

Thankfully, my dad went for a second opinion with oncologists at the Mayo Clinic in Jacksonville, Florida. Where the first oncologist gave my dad one treatment option, the Mayo Clinic gave another: a clinical trial for kidney cancer that was showing promising results. After some thought, my dad decided to enter the trial and hope for the treatment that could significantly extend his life. You don't always receive the experimental treatment when you enter a trial, but Dad's streak of luck continued and he was assigned the treatment—a combination of Avastin, a drug already on the market that disrupts the growth of blood vessels that would feed the cancer sites, and an experimental drug that helps stimulate the patient's own immune system to fight the cancer itself. Every three weeks, Dad would receive these drugs together with the hope of fighting back against the disease.

At his first scan after the treatment began, the tumors had begun to shrink. Today, over two years since beginning the treatment, Dad's tumors have shrunk by more than 50 percent. He continues to lead a normal life with minimal side effects. Dad is not dying from cancer, he is *living* with it. It is a manageable disease in the way that HIV/AIDS has become manageable. His oncologist has assured us that if Dad does die anytime soon, it will not be from cancer.

My family's introduction into the world of cancer has been a roller coaster of fear, hope, and the unknown. And unfortunately, we are not the only family to experience it. Millions of families will go through what my family has every year. And many of those families will not have as good of an outcome as mine has had. Why? Why can't we follow through on the promise made by generations of politicians to cure cancer? If nearly all of us will have experience with this dreaded disease either directly or indirectly in our lifetimes, why does it seem like we can do nothing about it? The answers to these and many other questions do not lie in the realm of science alone, or even hope or faith. Instead, there is a strong undercurrent of politics, social movements, and controversy that all affect the ways in which we study, view, and treat cancer.

It was my own training as a political scientist that prompted me to make these connections, although I did not originally set out to do so. I had started out my academic career studying space policy; I had also become engrossed in science policy in general, including environmental and budgetary politics. This naturally segued into asking the question what the government is doing or can do about things like cancer. Much to my surprise, or rather my chagrin, I found that many of the same problems that afflict something like human spaceflight also affect cancer research, from the start and stop of annual budgetary politics to embedded partisan issues. This is not to say that cancer policy in the United States is just like other science areas; it most certainly is not, if only because it is a topic that is likely to affect nearly all of us. Instead, these parallels have pushed me to think harder and deeper as to the barriers to effective cancer research and a lack of a cure since President Richard Nixon declared a war on cancer in 1971.

This book is, to the best of my knowledge, the first attempt to examine the politics of cancer from the perspective of a political scientist. Others have written a series of books and articles about it but from a scientific point of view. Although these scientist authors provide a valuable inside look at what they see as the Achilles' heel of cancer research and cancer policy, another perspective is certainly warranted. This book, in reviewing the political, social, scientific, and economic influences on U.S. cancer policy, argues that the way in which the American government conceives, creates, and carries out cancer policy is fundamentally flawed, inconsistent, and incoherent. No major policy actor, congressman, or president has taken a holistic view of all that is involved in cancer policy. It is not simply the money devoted to research and development or the organization of clinical trials, but the regulatory efforts at preventing cancer in the first place and the local politics that influence many of our politicians. It is the inconsistent and sub-jective nature of science itself, despite our beliefs that it should be inde-pendent and objective. It is the deep and embedded economic interests in our country that make pursuing further regulations incredibly difficult. It is our impatience with the scientists and what they do and do not know about cancer and our unrealistic high hopes for what can be done. In short, policy making in the United States is simply not conducive to making *good* policy, at least with respect to cancer.

In order to make this argument, this book takes an institutional per-spective in that it identifies the major political players in cancer policy and looks specifically at not only what those actors have or haven't done, but also what they can and cannot do, what limits their actions, and what motivates them. To better understand these behavioral impulses, this book adopts a political, social, scientific, and economic organizational framework; we uti-lize these four categories to analyze these different institutional actors and their behaviors, something that will be detailed in greater length in Chapter 2. And although this book most certainly speaks to the major actors in American politics such as the president and the Congress, it also goes into detail on the unsung actors, the bureaucracies, as well as public and eco-nomic interest groups. Without delving into these institutions, any expla-nation of how policy is made and implemented in the United States would be significantly lacking.

Chapter 1 begins with an introduction not only to cancer and the science behind it, but some of the major issues in research and development, including scientific pluralism, animal studies, and research methodology, as well as a look at government involvement in science and why government would be interested in science to begin with. Chapter 2 then introduces what we mean by political, social, scientific, and economic influences and sets the stage with a broad analysis of funding for the National Cancer Institute. As the government organization charged with leading the effort against cancer and the organization with the largest budget devoted to cancer research, understanding the dynamics through which the agency is funded can shed light on the actors discussed throughout the rest of the book.

Chapter 3 begins the institutional analysis of three of the most important bureaucracies in carrying out cancer policy: the Environmental Protection Agency, the National Cancer Institute, and the Food and Drug Administration. These three bureaucracies are variously charged with reducing our exposure to carcinogenic agents, making sure our food and drug supply is safe, and organizing the fight against cancer. Only then does Chapter 4 take up the issue of the president and the involvement of the executive office in the fight against cancer. This includes a look at how presidents have spoken about cancer and major policy statements made by presidents up through the "moon shot" effort against cancer launched by President Barack Obama and Vice President Joe Biden in 2016. Finally, Chapters 5 and 6 look at some of the most looming political actors, the Congress in Chapter 5 and public and private interest groups in Chapter 6. For all of the rhetoric about Congress's seeming lack of ability to do anything, they play a strong role in influencing not only budgets, but also how we view cancer and our public attention to it. Chapter 6's look at organized interests touches on some of the most controversial subjects in cancer policy, including the banning of tobacco (and the economic interests lined up against it), the cost of prescription drugs, and the power of the people to demand change.

Obviously, a book like this demands not only mental and academic effort but emotional perspective as well. To that end, it is practically impossible to call this work a solo effort, as I have received much encouragement and advice along the way. I would first like to thank my political science students at Cameron University who have patiently listened to early iterations of this "final" product. My wonderful colleagues in the Department of Social Sciences (formerly the Department of History and Government) also deserve thanks, most prominently Lance Janda, Sarah Janda, and Edris Montalvo.

Praeger editor Jessica Gribble is also deserving of my thanks; without her suggestion that this topic could be turned into a book, I probably would not have pursued this as early as I have. I certainly couldn't have done it as well without her thoughts and comments.

With a topic like cancer, family becomes the most important support of all. Thank you to my husband, Josh, whose job, once again, gave me time to complete this work. It was not just his job that gave me space and reason to work but also his never-failing support and love. Our animal "children," Gus and Bean, have also proven to be superior writing buddies when Bean isn't walking over the keyboard and Gus isn't barking to go outside.

My family, like many others who have confronted cancer, has become far closer as Dad has battled through. In the time since his second diagnosis, my sister welcomed the first granddaughter, Addison, to the fold, which has brightened everyone's outlook on life. And although there have been many life changes that have often been overwhelming, we've remained a tight-knit group who enjoys to laugh in the hardest of situations. We might not laugh right away, but eventually we will. Thank you to Mom, Grandmom, Jennifer, Sean, Addy, and Timmy.

Ultimately, if not about him directly, this book is for my Dad. It might not be the MBA you always wanted me to get, but I tend to think this is better in the end.

As always, all remaining errors are solely my own.

CHAPTER ONE

Introduction

The real terror of cancer is the silent, insidious nature of it. It is our body turning against itself, and we cannot reassert control over it. It quietly grows within us, and we are ignorant and helpless to stop it. Hardly a day goes by when we aren't told that something could cause cancer or something else could stop it. We're caught in a modern tug of war between the comforts and lifestyle of everyday living and the consequences it could have further down the road. Will drinking that cup of coffee or glass of wine help us prevent cancer or cause it? How much exercise do we need on a daily basis to reduce our chances of developing it? Are our desk jobs slowly killing us? The sheer anxiety is in thinking that something is slowly growing inside of you, entwining itself in the inner workings of the body, and living off of the very organs that keep you breathing, a dark force slowly suffocating your body to death.

In such panic-inducing scenarios, we look for help where we can. We first turn to our doctors to understand the nature and progression of the malevolent force using our body for its survival. The doctors use the tools at their disposal to diagnose and pinpoint the cause of the malady and discover how far it has advanced inside of us. We go to the specialists, those brave souls who have chosen to devote their life to battling back death, if only for a few days, weeks, months, and hopefully, years. The specialists delve into the science, the drugs, and the biology available to them to beat back the tumors. And when we have exhausted all available solutions and treatments, we grasp at those drugs and procedures that might offer some hope but may ultimately lead to death. We beg, borrow, and steal time from the cutting edge of science, holistic medicine, religion, faith, and even nihilism. And at the end, when there are no more Faustian bargains to be entered into, we shake our fists at the sky and cry for help from any arena that might be prepared to entertain such notions.

This includes crying to our governments and elected leaders for help. We beg those who have become servants of the people to do what they can to alleviate our suffering. Provide the tools and resources to treat—if not cure—this disease of extended life and modern living. They protect us from so many other dangers, why not cancer? Why shouldn't our government do everything in its power to save us, even if it's not something we originally envisioned as something a government would do or could do? This is how cancer, a disease so often unseen, becomes a political football to be kicked, thrown, deflated, and promoted all at the same time. A rhetorical call to arms, politicians have taken up the mantle, adopting the calls to end cancer as their own and initiating a process that government is simply not capable of fully carrying out.

This book represents an attempt at understanding the political dynamics of cancer policy in the United States. The highly personal nature of the disease is counterposed by the highly political nature of its treatment. Although the millions of Americans afflicted by cancer (along with their families and friends) may not realize it, how we understand and treat cancer is not something that is driven by science and medicine but by political, social, scientific, and economic understandings of cancer and how to treat it. In addition to the unfairness of the disease and how it strikes us, we add the unfairness of the political system and add insult upon injury in making cancer the political football that it has become.

In many ways, the fact that cancer has become political is an inevitable consequence of the growth of modern democratic government. As government has historically moved to prevent its citizens from experiencing the harms of living, government intrusion into medicine, disease, and ultimately cancer naturally flows from this pattern of growth. The increase of the regulatory state that ensures that the drugs and food that we take and eat are safe leads us to question what safety ultimately is. Regulating and licensing medical professionals to ensure that they have the requisite education, understanding, and training in medicine puts an official stamp on those who practice the medical arts. In providing medical care and insurance to the elderly and those less fortunate, the government puts its imprimatur on the types of treatments and drugs that it will cover, thereby legitimizing certain treatments over others. Government support in the form of research dollars supports certain types of research over others, pruning at the root the types of studies and research that will be carried out and understood. These and many other aspects of government control are all involved in the treatment and understanding of cancer today.

While there has been widespread acknowledgement of this situation from political scientists to historians, from scientists to politicians, there has been no in-depth study of cancer as a whole and the politics involved in it. In the grand scheme of history, this acknowledgement is a very recent one, coinciding with a societal recognition that cancer is a growing and malicious problem. To better understand how this situation has evolved and come to be, this chapter will lay out not only the briefest outline of the history of cancer, but also an exploration of some of the major themes in the confluence of cancer and politics. These themes greatly influence how political actors deal with cancer policy in the United States, and it is the interactions among these actors that create cancer policy in the United States.

A Brief History of Cancer

An excellent treatment of the subject is available in Siddhartha Mukherjee's *The Emperor of All Maladies: A Biography of Cancer* so I will not recount the history in full. Although cancer has most likely been around for as long as humans have walked the earth, the history of cancer is really comparatively brief. Along with archaeological evidence of sarcomas (bone cancer), the earliest historical description of cancer comes from an Egyptian papyrus from around the 17th century CE that contains the medical teachings of Imhotep, an advisor to the pharaohs.[1] In the papyrus, Imhotep describes tumors of the breast and says that there are no treatments for them and "[w]ith that admission of impotence, cancer virtually disappeared from ancient medical history."[2] Later descriptions of the disease from ancient Greece onward drew on the medical understandings available to physicians of the day, primarily the theory that illness in the body emanated from the four humors (blood, yellow bile, black bile, and phlegm) being out of balance. Based on this belief, treatment for tumors was limited to surgical (and therefore painful) excision or bloodletting to supposedly rebalance the essential components of the body.

This understanding of illness and medicine persisted into the period of the scientific enlightenment beginning in the 17th century. However, the incidence of cancer relative to other, more persistent diseases was relatively low. People were more likely to die of the plague, yellow fever, smallpox, or any other number of epidemics than they were to die of cancer. As medical knowledge slowly began to advance and accumulate, particularly in the 1800s, beliefs about cancer began to change. Marie and Pierre Curie's research into radiation led not only to the realization that radiation could cause cancer, but to the knowledge that it could be used to treat it as well.

Other scientists were able to identify dangerous chemicals as potentially cancer-causing agents. Even research into chickens and viruses at the turn of the 20th century suggested a viral cause of cancer. The advancement of surgical techniques and technology, including the advent of anesthesia, led to radical surgeries, particularly in the case of breast cancer, to alleviate suffering.

Moving into the 20th century, as scientists and doctors were beginning to better understand and treat cancer, socially it was treated carefully and quietly. Cancer was not often discussed; it was something to be hidden, to be ashamed of. The private nature of the disease can be contrasted with the more public events that would contribute to the growth of cancer incidence and study. While people were suffering in silence, the advances of the 20th century in war, technology, politics, and science were coming together to promote a disease that was far more private than public. Indeed, it is easy to understand why cancer, when compared to other diseases and afflictions, was dealt with more in private than in public. Often, there are no outward physical signs or symptoms that signal someone is suffering from cancer; in contrast, polio can leave children paralyzed, and smallpox can leave you scarred. These physical ailments lead to a more public understanding of the diseases compared to those we suffer in private.

What were these events that would bring cancer to the forefront of our concerns, of our lives? Scientifically and technologically, medical advances were coming fast and quick. Using new technology, scientists could look through a microscope at the tissues and cells that make up our body and for the first time see what was happening at a cellular level. Doctors could see and compare cancer cells with healthy cells to aid in diagnosis and treatment of cancer. They could understand for the first time that cancer cells were the body's own cells turned into reproduction machines with no off switch. Military advancements aided the cause. While the use of mustard gas in the trenches of World War I left thousands of soldiers dead, scientists also noted the effect that mustard gas had on cancerous tumors, helping to lead to the development of chemotherapy whereby cancer could be treated via the administration of particular drugs. Military developments continued through to World War II. With the establishment of the Manhattan Project, government needed to know not only the effects of radiation on a large scale, but also on a small one. Both of these military advancements contributed to cancer research and treatment well into the mid-20th century in providing funding for research and setting an example of large-scale, industrial-style science.

Other scientific advancements naturally led to a greater focus on cancer. The creation of the Salk vaccine for polio and the development of penicillin led to cures or treatment for some of society's most feared diseases. Life expectancies correspondingly increased, and as people led longer lives, there was a greater chance for cancer to develop and cause death rather than the diseases that had traditionally ended people's lives. The success of the March of Dimes movement in generating the funding for research that led to the polio vaccine also provided a model for those interested in researching cancer to generate and develop support for a sustained effort against the disease.

Many of these trends came together in a hospital in Boston in the 1940s. Dr. Sidney Farber, a pathologist at Boston Children's Hospital, specialized in studying cancers in children, particularly leukemia. Leukemia, cancer of the blood, was practically a death sentence at this point in time, but using the emerging science of the day, Farber sought out drugs that would attack the cancerous cells, but unfortunately destroying the bodies of the most helpless victims. Mukherjee describes childhood leukemia at the time as "the oddest and most hopeless variant" of all the cancers.[3] After finding that folic acid contributed to the explosive growth of cancer cells, Farber turned to antifolates, reasoning that if folic acid sped the growth of cancer, antifolates would slow it. Surprisingly, the antifolate aminopterin was found to be successful in arresting (at least temporarily) the spread of leukemia in a child, providing at least some hope that successful treatments could be found.

Farber's trials and errors with chemotherapy for childhood leukemia continued throughout the 1950s. At the same time, charity groups, inspired by the success of the March of Dimes, began to look for another disease on which to focus the public's attention. Out of this began the Jimmy Fund, which centered on Farber's Children's Hospital in Boston, and the newly renamed American Cancer Society (ACS), with its influential and politically savvy socialite, Mary Lasker. The Jimmy Fund supported the expansion of Boston Children's Hospital, and Mary Lasker's ACS grabbed hold of Farber's developments and used Farber, a trusted doctor, as the spokesperson for emerging cancer research. The fact that Farber's research was focused on children didn't hurt either; the face of the cancer epidemic became the innocent, vulnerable face of a child affected by leukemia, something their little bodies were helpless against. All of these trends led to an increased attention to cancer, including most importantly of all, political attention.

Early political attention on cancer really began in the early part of the 20th century with congressional policy entrepreneurs seeking ways to encourage the study of cancer. By 1937, the National Cancer Institute (NCI) was legislatively established to provide a central guiding force in the research of cancer. This represented the first time that the U.S. government provided funding and support for a noncommunicable disease, demonstrating the early political support for cancer research. It also occurred as concern over cancer reached a high point in the 1930s; funding for cancer research rose 24-fold between 1937 and 1951.[4] Throughout this period, the entire political establishment demonstrated growing interest in cancer (to be explored in more depth in later chapters), connecting it to issues as varied as social security, polio, health care reform, and Medicaid and Medicare. At the same time, presidential interest grew, peaking with Lyndon B. Johnson in the 1960s.

Why Johnson in the 1960s? Mary Lasker, as the de facto head of the American Cancer Society, was not only an effective organizer but a political force to be reckoned with. Lasker had cultivated political relationships for years, and her relationship with Johnson stretched back to Johnson's time in the U.S. Senate. Johnson's focus on cancer as an issue is demonstrated in the increasing number of statements he made about cancer while he was president. Mukherjee also details Lasker's significant relationship with Johnson, and the fact that bureaucratic agencies took her and her organization seriously is reflective of the influence that Lasker had on LBJ. Throughout this period, Lasker and the ACS had begun to call for an all-out assault on cancer, which would finally find its champion not in Johnson but in Richard Nixon.

Lasker continued her assault on presidential thought early in Nixon's presidency; one of the tactics the ACS adopted was taking out a full-page ad in *The New York Times* calling for Nixon to declare a war on cancer. The campaign worked, and in the 1970 State of the Union, Nixon asked for over $100 million in funding for the war on cancer. The end result was the National Cancer Act of 1971, which not only granted a large influx of funds for cancer research, but also granted expanded powers to the NCI and the National Institutes of Health (NIH) to organize and direct cancer research. This governmental backing would belie the scientific reality that there was no scientific consensus on the best ways to tackle the cancer epidemic or even what cancer was caused by. It's hard to imagine, but even as late as the 1970s, researchers still did not understand the underlying mechanisms of carcinogenesis, or what causes a perfectly healthy and normal cell to turn to the dark side and become cancer.

Scientific uncertainty centered around two major foci: the causes of cancer (carcinogenesis) and whether researchers should pursue prevention or treatment of cancer as their main goal. To begin with carcinogenesis, scientists understood that in order to be able to treat and eventually cure cancer, they would need to know just what causes cancer in the first place. To this point, there had been three major theories as to what causes carcinogenesis: environmental factors, genetic factors, and viral factors. With respect to viruses, we now recognize today that human papilloma virus (HPV) can cause a number of cancers, including cervical and some throat and oral cancers. However, the viral argument for cancer has its origins in the 1910s and 1920s with the research of Peyton Rous, who studied sarcomas in chickens.[5] Rous concluded that a particular type of sarcoma in chickens, spindle-cell sarcoma, was in fact caused by a virus that would come to be named the Rous sarcoma virus.[6] Although there was scant evidence beyond HPV that there were any viruses that actually led to cancer, by the 1960s, "the cancer virus theory was in full spate—in part because viruses were the new rage in all medicine."[7] The idea that cancer was something that we could catch, and therefore prevent, stoked the public imagination with promises of potential treatments and even cures.

The burgeoning field of genomics coming on the heels of the discovery of DNA in 1953 offered yet another route to carcinogenesis. The fact that some cancers appeared to be hereditary provided researchers an opportunity to study genetic changes that might correspond with the incidence of cancer. However, many scientists were potentially put off from such studies because of the possible connections to eugenics and the recent Nazi ideology that emphasized the extermination of those deemed inferior; if cancer's roots lie in an individual's genes, then perhaps there would be those who would want to rid the human population of such defects. As science and medicine advanced and we moved further away from the terror and tragedies of World War II, greater genetic study became yet another avenue for cancer researchers to exploit.

With respect to environmental factors, in the early 1900s, there were known environmental carcinogens, including radiation and "organic chemicals, such as paraffin and dye by-products" as well as chimney soot and smoke.[8] By the time of Nixon's declaration of war, the environmental movement had identified many other chemicals as potentially harmful to humans and even carcinogenic. Those who advocated for an environmental cause to cancer argued that the best way to treat it was to prevent it in the first place by outlawing cancer-causing environmental agents.

The dispute about environmental causes of cancer directly led to the second controversy in cancer policy: either work to prevent cancer from forming by addressing environmental and viral causes of cancer, or focus on researching treatments and possible cures for cancer. Brown and colleagues describe the difference between treatment and prevention this way:

> Primary prevention (upstream) emphasizes disease prevention in populations. In an environmental health context, this includes strategies aimed at

preventing human exposure to toxics through pollution prevention and toxic-use reduction. Secondary prevention aims to provide screening, early detection of disease, and prompt intervention for people at risk for disease. Tertiary prevention (downstream) minimizes the effect of disease in people who are already quite sick . . . A walk upstream implies a radical shift in research and intervention away from tertiary approaches such as treatment efficacy (surgery, radiation, and pharmacological treatments) and secondary prevention such as screening and early detection . . . and toward minimizing exposures to risk factors and toxic substances that may be linked to disease.[9]

Particularly in the afterglow of the environmental movement and the recognition that smoking does indeed cause cancer, many activists and researchers insisted that the proper way to deal with the cancer epidemic was to get rid of the environmental causes. This perspective adopts the rationale that cancer is preventable, that it is not inevitable that any one individual should get cancer. A number of prominent cancer researchers were critical of the lack of attention the cancer establishment gave to prevention. During the 1960s, Wilhelm Hueper, an official within the NCI, was openly critical of the lack of prevention efforts, believing that the vast majority of cancer cases could be prevented.[10] However, Hueper was widely derided by the cancer establishment and his views largely ignored.[11] Efforts at identifying pollutants continued into the 1970s when Samuel Epstein, another cancer researcher, claimed that industrial pollutants and other chemicals were largely responsible for cancer cases and that industry and government were conspiring to cover up the relationships.[12] The debate between environmental causes and the avenue of prevention versus treatment of cancer is an example of how dominant paradigms or beliefs about the nature of cancer worked against minority researchers to stifle possibly compelling evidence and limit examination of controversial topics. The essential point, however, is that despite the increased funding and attention, there was no scientific agreement on an approach to studying cancer. The war on cancer would never be able to be a concerted effort dedicated toward one enemy; instead the resources and the army would be split in contradictory directions.

Since the 1970s, the rhetoric of the war on cancer continues to be invoked by politicians of all stripes, while our understanding of cancer has undoubtedly been advanced. Today, we understand the origins of carcinogenesis lie in the faulty genes that regulate, or fail to regulate in the case of cancer, the replication of cells. Whether these oncogenes, the genes that are responsible for the unfettered replication, are triggered by environment or viruses, or are inherent in an individual's genetic code, DNA is at the heart of carcinogenesis. Scientists have even been able to identify some of these faulty genes such as BRCA1 and BRCA2 in the case of breast cancer. Researchers have developed targeted treatments and begun to focus on immunotherapy to harness the power of an individual's own immune system to destroy cancerous cells. These advancements, however, disguise the criticism that the war on cancer has failed, that people are still dying, and that the ever elusive cure has yet to be found.

Since the 1980s, whether we're winning or losing the war on cancer has itself become a political hotbed of controversy. Particularly given that government funds have been devoted to cancer research, politicians must show that their programs and policies are working; can the war on cancer be said to be successful? Now some 45 years removed from the beginning of the war on cancer, some critics have seen little advancement in the search for a cure.[13] Although the number of cancer survivors has risen, so has the realization that cancer is not a single ailment but multiple, each responding (or not) to different treatments.[14] This debate is similarly difficult to answer because just as scientists looking at the same data can come to wildly different conclusions, depending on the statistics and methodology you use to measure success against cancer, both proponents and opponents of the war on cancer can summon data that supports their arguments. The complicated field of epidemiology, the study of patterns of health and illness, has at its fingertips a mass of data on people who live, die, suffer, and are exposed. Depending on how these statistics are sliced and diced, scientists can argue that the number of cancer deaths has declined or increased. The epidemiologists themselves became the subject of political attention; Devra Davis, a former NIH epidemiologist, describes in detail her experience with cancer statistics in *The Secret History of the War on Cancer*. Davis describes how "[t]he PR flacks made me out to be a deluded zealot" over the epidemiological statistics in order to undermine her effectiveness in guiding the Clinton administration's breast cancer policy.[15] The great debate of the politics of cancer thus became what effect the investment in cancer research was or wasn't having.

What most everyone can agree on, now some 45 years after Nixon's original declaration of war, is that we have made progress in our knowledge of cancer from carcinogenesis to its treatments. Is it the type of progress that Lasker and other early cancer activists and researchers had hoped for or expected? The answer is decidedly no. Are people still suffering from cancer? Yes, but treatment has advanced far beyond the rudimentary chemotherapy techniques available in 1971. Is the war won in the sense that we have cured cancer? No, but we're not losing either.

At the Intersection of Government and Science

In order to truly understand the nature of the relationship between government and science, we need to ask the following questions: Why is government getting involved in science and why is science interested in government? There is no mention in the Constitution of science, research, or medicine and no provisions through which government can participate in science. Why would the U.S. government, let alone any government, involve itself in such an area when there are many other concerns that governments should be involved in? In a set of reflections about this very confluence, cancer researcher Salvador Luria argues that "[o]ur society is fundamentally based on the premise of democracy. Modern democracy is the daughter of the rationalism of the seventeenth and eighteenth centuries and is therefore in a sense the twin sister of science."[16] What Luria is referring to is the influence of the Enlightenment on both science and government; a period of new philosophical thinking about both science and government, the Enlightenment introduced a sense of rationality, purpose, and method to both fields. Commitment to scientific principles based on experimentation and study rather than faith and religion ran parallel to the rejection of the divine right of kings and the acknowledgement of natural rights, social contracts, and constitutionally based republics like the United States. Yet although science and government developed similarly at the same point in time, this does not necessarily mean that the two were destined to intertwine and find themselves in a symbiotic relationship.

Theoretically, pure government, the act of governing a state, does not need science; that is, they don't until they do. In the United States, the utilization of science and the fostering of research and development came about slowly as the need arose. The oldest regulatory body in the United States, the Food and Drug Administration (FDA), has its roots in the antebellum period when the Patent Office undertook a program to study agricultural products. This office was transferred to the newly formed Department of Agriculture under Abraham Lincoln, and its powers and purpose have grown ever since, particularly in the Progressive Era. Progressive activists at the turn of the 20th century recognized a number of societal ills that they believed government could be used to solve, including childhood labor, unsafe working conditions, and the health and safety of food and drugs in the United States. When the 1906 Pure Food and Drug Act was passed, the government claimed a role in regulating food and drugs to ensure the safety of its people. In order to perform such activities, government was necessarily invoking science in order to inform their decisions. The modern regulatory state has only grown since, and it implicitly relies on science for information and data on which to base its decisions on everything from regulating cancer-causing chemicals to medical technology.

Government fostering of medical research was also established at this time with the creation of the National Board of Health in 1887. This new agency was given funding to research deadly communicable diseases like cholera and yellow fever. In the same year, the Quarantine Act was passed enabling local governments to proactively move to abet possible epidemics that would cause public harm. These early programs coalesced into the Public Health Service by 1910, and in 1930 the National Institutes of Health was created. This pattern of development demonstrates government interest in ensuring the health and safety of its population and reinforced the role of government in doing so.

At the same time as the Progressive movement was developing and asserting its will, there was a concurrent movement for rationality and scientifically based principles in government itself. In the late 1800s, political science was established as an academic field not only to study the development of the state and politics, but also as a rational, scientific influence on the form and functioning of government itself. Woodrow Wilson, one of the earliest political scientists and later president, wrote in 1887, "I suppose that no practical science is ever studied where there is no need to know it. The very fact, therefore, that the eminently practical science of administration is finding its way into college courses in this country would prove that this country needs to know more about administration."[17] Wilson was making the argument that through scientific study of policy and administration, political scientists could contribute to a better functioning of government by providing advice and ideas to policy makers that were discovered in the course of fact-based research. "It is the object of administrative study to discover, first, what government can properly and successfully do, and secondly, how it can do these proper things with the utmost possible efficiency and at the least possible cost either of money or energy."[18]

By the turn of the 20th century, science and government were becoming more closely intertwined and the pace of interaction only increased. Countries around the world, including the United States, were quickly realizing that they could use scientific advancements to their advantage, both economically and militarily. World War I ushered in a new era of military technology in terms of chemical weapons and air combat; the period between World War I and World War II hastened this relationship, with the Manhattan Project being the ultimate example of government using science to their advantage. Military research and development continued after World War II, and government soon realized that technological spin-offs could be beneficial economically as well as militarily. The space race and its

attendant technology stemmed from missile and rocket technology originally developed by the military and would go on to produce innumerable
economic benefits not only the 1960s but continuing today.

Throughout the 20th century, the growth of the regulatory state continued, government interest was established in looking after public health
and the food and drug supply, and government support for scientific research
and development increased markedly. The intertwining of science and government did not occur haphazardly; relationships were established in areas
of government need, and the result is that government tends to promote
the science it can expect to benefit from. After all, the government benefits
when its populace is healthy and able to produce economically. But what
does science get out of this relationship? Is it a one-way road or a mutually
beneficial relationship?

Unfortunately, science needs more than good ideas and knowledge to
be successful. The underpinning of the scientific and medical establishment
is that knowledge is derived from experimentation and study; it is those
activities that are often incredibly costly to undertake. Physical facilities,
laboratory equipment, and research assistants are all required to complete
successful experiments, and all of those requirements cost money. Many
scientists and researchers today can draw on the resources they get from
the academic community; universities and other educational facilities provide scientists with the needed resources to undertake their desired activities. However, the amount of money that many of these universities have
access to is often limited and dedicated to other educational activities.
Especially in an era like today where the costs of a modern university are
rising, there have been severe limits to the amount of money that can be
dedicated to research and development, forcing scientists to look elsewhere
for monetary support. With a swelling federal budget and more need for
scientific expertise, the federal government has become a valuable source
of funding for scientific endeavors. Science, therefore, needs government
for the support and resources it can provide.

And there are some things that only the government can fund. Massive
research undertakings that cost big dollars can really only be supported
by government. The space program is only one example of a scientific
endeavor that costs more money than the private sector could collectively
provide. In addition to human spaceflight, the government has contributed
to the construction and operation of major observatories like the Arecibo
radio telescope in Puerto Rico and the Very Large Array operated by
the National Radio Astronomy Observatory. This doesn't mean that it was
always easy for large science projects to receive government funding; the
Superconducting Super Collider, a planned particle accelerator in Texas,

had its funding canceled in 1993. Prior to cancellation, over $2 billion was spent on the project, but the program was a victim of the ever-increasing cost estimates being provided.

The resources government has and can provide are significant. Even after peaking in the mid-1960s and slowly declining since, the amount of money dedicated in 2016 to nondefense research and development is over $67 billion.[19] When military research and development is included in that, the total amount rises to $143 billion.[20] With such dollars available to researchers, it's only natural that they should turn to government looking for support. In fact, government grant dollars have become so intrinsic to the academic community that tenure and promotion decisions for academic scientists will take into consideration just how much grant money a professor has brought to the school. Thus, academic researchers have an even greater incentive to pursue government research and development dollars.

However plentiful the money may appear to be, it's not handed out to just anybody. What does it take to get that government support? Quite simply, you pursue the science that's most likely to get the money. An excellent example of this problem is military research into the effects of low-level radiation in the 1940s and 1950s. Gerald Kutcher details the sometimes insidious relationship between military and medical research, in this case, cancer research. With the Manhattan Project underway in the 1940s, the military soon found that they needed to know what effects, if any, long-term, low-dose radiation exposure would have on individuals. This need only increased following Hiroshima and Nagasaki and the advent of possible nuclear war during the Cold War. Funding for radiation studies soon flowed not only from the National Cancer Institute but from the Atomic Energy Commission and the Department of Defense.[21] Cancer researchers such as Donnall Thomas and Eugene Saenger benefitted from the military funding, performing experiments that exposed the sickest cancer patients to low levels of radiation. What was most insidious about these trials is that the researchers would claim that patients were exposed to systemic low-level radiation in order to treat their cancer when the real purpose was military research into the effects of the radiation.[22] Kutcher therefore argues that "researchers adjust their investigations to draw on the available epistemological, material, and monetary resources" available to them.

When looked at holistically, it would appear that this situation is win-win; science gets the money and resources that it needs, and government gets the information it wants. However, when looked at from a different angle, the conclusion can be different. If the only approved type of science to be studied or performed is the science desired by government, some legitimate science may be ignored or never pursued. This problem relates back to the nature of the scientific establishment itself; despite the appearance of mass scientific agreement on certain procedures or applications of the knowledge gained, the appearance of agreement masks sometimes sharp disagreements among researchers themselves. If a researcher seems to be on a fortuitous line of study but that approach is not recognized as legitimate or worthy of study, the researcher may be denied the funds, resources, and ability to pursue such experimentation. Potentially fruitful lines of research may be abandoned before we fully know what they might be capable of. If the receipt of government funding is a signal that the research performed is legitimate and useful, the nonreceipt of funding can equally be interpreted as a sign of lack of promise.

And the decision of what science to fund is an inherently political question. To demonstrate this, we need look only at the criticisms of the politicians themselves like former Senator William Proxmire (D-WI). In 1975, Proxmire began to issue monthly "Golden Fleece Awards" to scientists and other government programs that he believed were "wasting" federal tax dollars. A prime example of the types of studies the Golden Fleece Awards were directed toward was one National Science Foundation (NSF) grant in 1975 to study how people fall in love.[23] Proxmire's intent on publicizing such ventures was to shame the government into not providing the funds to such "useless" or "wasteful" ventures. But who's to say what is useless or wasteful? Even the study on falling in love could provide valuable insights as to the workings of the human brain. Another example of how political science funding can be involves political science itself. Beginning in 2009, Senator Tom Coburn (R-OK) called for ending the $5 million in NSF funding that is directed toward political science research, calling it wasteful.[24] Coburn was finally successful in 2014 in eliminating political science research funding, although those funds were restored in 2015. Although the politics of science funding will be discussed more fully, it is sufficient here to recognize that not funding certain research avenues while funding others essentially leaves government in the role of determining what is legitimate science and what is not, something that deeply affects cancer policy.

Part of the criticism leveled at such "Golden Fleece" funding recipients is that it is often difficult to defend government funding that does not lead to some direct benefit. Particularly in an age where great attention is leveled at the government budget and budgeting shortfalls, politicians often want and need results from funded studies to justify the spending decisions. It is much harder to defend funding a research project that may have no tangible benefits or conclusion than it is to defend funding a project that has a direct impact on the lives of Americans. Therefore, government funds are often targeted to certain kinds of applied science rather than basic research. It is far easier to call for a cure for cancer than a better under-standing of it. This is yet another way that government funding discrimi-nates among scientific pursuits and systematically discourages other studies such as basic research into the nature of carcinogenesis.

The reason that there is often significant conflict between the needs of the scientists and the politicians is because in each profession there exist different motivations for their behavior. What's more, these motivations very often conflict. An elected official, by definition, is reliant on his or her voters for their job; political science readily recognizes this electoral incen-tive as a key driver of political behavior.[25] If elected officials do not seem-ingly respond to the wishes and desires of their constituents, they will soon find themselves out of a job. As such, politicians have a strong desire to respond not only to crisis, but show their constituents progress in policy making. This makes the war on cancer a very attractive rhetorical propo-sition for policy makers since it is quite likely that their constituents will have some experience with the dreaded disease.

Scientists do experience a similar pressure of needing to be responsive to a particular group of individuals. However, in this case, the group that they often seek to please, at least in the world of academia, is other scien-tists. In academics, the way in which professors find themselves advanced is primarily through the publication of research in peer-reviewed journals. Because other scientists must approve of the publication before it appears in print, a large amount of pressure is put on academic scientists to perform and publish the research that will likely find legitimacy and credibility from other mainstream scientists. "Scientists who follow the dominant approach" to research in a field "have a greater ability to obtain research funding, scientific prestige, and career advancement."[26] There is no pres-sure to show that their findings have or will have a relevance or that there is a cost/benefit equation involved. This differs from the political pressure of demonstrating need, relevance, and financial responsibility for fear of being issued a Golden Fleece award or having to field questions from fellow members of Congress and constituents about the need for certain studies.

These differences between scientists and politicians also reflect the dif-ferences between policy and science. Sheila Jasanoff, in exploring how the Environmental Protection Agency (EPA) has developed and sustained policies against carcinogenic products, argues that the

> . . . development of guidelines for assessing cancer risks seems in retro-spect to have stood the normal process of scientific fact making on its head. The reason becomes clear if we compare EPA's objectives and strategies in risk assessment with those of ordinary working scientists who seek to

translate laboratory observations into factual claims. . . . The successful scientist makes claims that become so routine and so indispensable that no one stops to question them or to probe into the circumstances behind their making. . . .

In the context of regulation, by contrast, scientific "facts" serve as a bridge not to other facts but to policy decisions. They undergo no subsequent testing at the hands of scientists, so that their legitimacy depends exclusively on the manner of their production.[27]

In other words, scientific understanding and discovery depend on continued testing and evaluation, whereas policy making depends on the process used to get there, not necessarily the information it stands on. Whereas scientific disputes can be settled by repeated tests, research, and the scientific community, political disputes are not usually settled that rationally.

Scientific Pluralism: Risk and Uncertainty

As previously mentioned, "science" is not monolithic; very often disagreements emerge not only over the interpretation of data but over the data itself. When the scientific community can't even agree on an approach to researching or treating ailments like cancer, this can have a significant effect not only on the research carried out, but also on how the political community reacts to such disagreements. This point was dramatically brought home in a 2015 study that attempted to replicate the findings of 100 psychological studies from 2008 onward.[28] In trying to replicate these findings, the authors found that up to half of the findings could not be re-created by the authors despite using the original experimental setups. If one of the hallmarks of "good" science is the ability to replicate results to ensure validity, what does it say about the state of research when this can't be done?

There are a number of areas in scientific research where scientists do not necessarily agree, and this uncertainty directly affects research into cancer and the policy emerging out of it. These areas include aspects of experimental methodology, the appropriateness of animal studies, and ideas about risk and appropriate levels of risk. To understand the uncertainty involved in each of these aspects, we can review how they have been involved in actual cancer research.

Animal Studies

A spate of studies have examined an intriguing question: despite access to the same data on possible carcinogenic elements, why do different countries come to different conclusions about how and if they should be regulated? Two such debates relate to cancer research: estrogen replacement therapy and the pesticide aldrin/dieldrin (A/D). Despite evidence that both cause cancer, the United States and Great Britain came to different conclusions about whether they should be used or not. In the case of A/D, there existed correlations between human exposure to the pesticide and cancer, but only a small population of individuals had been consistently exposed to it for more than 10 years.[29] What direct evidence did exist were animal-based studies that exposed laboratory animals to A/D; Shell, the maker of A/D, argued that animal studies are not indicative of how humans react to the chemical. This is a common critique of animal-based studies, with many arguing that just because a chemical causes cancer in a mouse or rat does not mean that it will cause cancer in humans. Not only do mice and humans have different physiological structures, the mice are exposed to massive doses of the suspected carcinogen, doses that humans likely would never be exposed to. In hearings before the EPA on whether the license to use A/D should be suspended or not, Shell made ample use of this argument.[30]

Critics of the animal experiment point to a number of factors that differentiate animal tests from human tests. First, as Shell argued in the case of A/D, mice are unsuitable for study because they are quite sensitive to chemicals and are known to spontaneously grow tumors.[31] Second, the tests that mice are subjected to are simplistic in nature; where the mice might only be exposed to one chemical at a time, in reality, humans are bombarded with many different chemicals all at the same time. The potential interactions of different chemicals could lead to different results in humans.[32] Third, animals are usually subjected to large amounts of chemicals, far larger than the amounts that humans are typically exposed to. And finally, animal tests are usually short term, whereas human exposures happen over long periods.

Clearly, there are problems with animal studies; however, proponents will argue that the alternative would be to experiment on humans, something that is not only unethical but clearly unacceptable. Further, they counter that animals such as mice have shorter life spans, necessitating the administration of large doses of chemicals and allowing for short-term studies. Short-term studies are also essential, they would say, because otherwise we could go our entire lives being exposed to a chemical, never knowing whether it is causing a growing monster inside of us.

In sum, although there are problems with animal studies, they are really the only feasible option in studying carcinogenic, or possibly carcinogenic, materials. Realizing the drawbacks, scientists know that demonstrating toxicity in animals is only a precursor to possible human harm; nobody is solely relying on them to make conclusions or decisions but they can serve as early warnings. In fact, scientists, along with pharmaceutical companies, have been intensely involved in developing new animal models and establishing standards for determining carcinogenicity in mice.[33]

Experimental Methodology

The classic and most basic form of the scientific experiment involves two groups: an experimental group and a control group. A treatment is given to the experimental group with either nothing or a placebo being given to the other; the results are then compared to see what the effect of the treatment was compared to the control group. However, in practice, experimental methodology can be quite a bit more complex. How many people do you need to include in the experimental and control groups? Do they need to be healthy or sick? Are you comparing the effects of the treatment to a control group that gets no treatment or to another group that gets a different treatment? How much of a response to the treatment is needed in order to declare that it works? What if only one person responds to the treatment and no one else? These are questions that the scientific establishment has wrestled over for decades.[34]

These types of questions were involved in questions over the effectiveness of vitamin C in fighting cancer. The use of vitamin C in treating cancer was advocated by two scientists: Nobel winner Linus Pauling and Ewan Cameron.[35] In the 1970s, Cameron administered this vitamin C treatment to more than 500 terminal cancer patients and found that the treatment, although not curing cancer, did provide some beneficial effects to patients, including the alleviation of symptoms and side effects of traditional drugs and some shrinkage of tumors.[36] Given that this initial study was uncontrolled, the rest of the scientific establishment did not put much credence in the findings. As a result, Cameron proceeded with a second study that compared a group of 100 terminal patients with matched control cases found in hospital records; this study showed that the experimental group survived 210 days compared to the control group.[37] Still, other scientists did not believe the findings because the groups were not randomized, a key aspect of experimental studies to reduce the amount of random error that might be involved.

Ultimately, the controversy over vitamin C led the National Cancer Institute to fund a study at the Mayo Clinic that would be controlled and randomized; this study concluded that there were no benefits to vitamin C therapy. But just as Cameron's study came in for criticism by the scientific community, Cameron and Pauling roundly criticized the methodology of the Mayo Clinic study. "The major difference was that, by contrast with Cameron's patients, most of the Mayo Clinic patients had had prior chemotherapy which, Pauling and Cameron claimed, had so weakened their immune systems as to negate the benefits to be obtained from vitamin C."[38] The Mayo administrators claimed that it would have been unethical to only administer vitamin C, a drug with unknown benefit, instead of chemotherapy, a drug with known effectiveness. The result was a second Mayo study with vitamin C administered to patients who had not yet received chemotherapy; the results were the same as before: no effect.

The vitamin C incident demonstrates that the methodology by which scientists undertake their studies is easily and often disputed. Added together with the role of replication (or the inability to replicate as noted earlier), it is easy to understand how even scientists themselves may be unsure of the results that they get in their research. In fact, criticisms of methodology don't just affect areas like cancer research, but are key arguments in opponents of global warming, who claim that the way we study climate is uncertain and unsure.

Levels of Risk and Uncertainty

When scientists seek to interpret the body of work and findings in a field, they must weigh two categories: standards of proof and weight of evidence.[39] Standards of proof "are the norms with which research is interpreted," and there are often disputes over just what these norms are.[40] These standards include things of the type that we have just discussed: scientific methodology and the use of animal studies. The fact that different norms can be considered is evidence that science is not as neutral and value free as we have been led to believe; depending on an individual scientist's belief about what constitutes the "standard," the findings of various studies can be interpreted in different ways. Similarly, the weight of evidence involves the determination of the broad conclusions that can be taken from a group of studies, but there are also disputes over what studies should be included and whether negative findings should be considered.[41] These elements of uncertainty in the science on which policy is eventually based lead to far more problems than can initially be seen.

Gillespie, Eva, and Johnston, in their study of A/D, conclude that the EPA and British authorities used different standards to determine whether A/D causes cancer or not, with the most immediate difference being the interpretation of the evidence provided. British regulators did not believe that the risk rose to a high enough level to warrant banning A/D, whereas the EPA did believe the risk was substantial enough. The case of A/D is not the only one in which this pattern held; different conclusions were also reached in the case of estrogen replacement therapy. McCrea and Markle note that "American and British researchers have evolved different criteria which are necessary to impute carcinogenicity," with British work being far more conservative and more reluctant to declare something carcinogenic than American research.[42] "The British demand evidence of causality before a substance is judged carcinogenic; in the US a demonstrated risk, as determined by scientific consensus is sufficient."[43] The scientific community, then, does have different standards of significance; if researchers can't agree on the evidence that makes something carcinogenic, how can policy makers take action on it?

"Science itself, the nature of scientific knowledge, and the habitual ways in which scientists couch their judgments—e.g., the language of uncertainty, probability, tentativeness—have become powerful tools in the political fights over health and safety regulation."[44] Science, by its very nature, is inherently uncertain. When studies do not include the entire human population (which are necessarily all of them), they must use inferential statistics which allows for random error to be involved; results are reported within a confidence interval which specifically requires a certain level of uncertainty into the results. This is where replicability of findings becomes so important; replicated studies provide a greater level of certainty. However, this required element of uncertainty can lead to real political and health consequences in cancer research and policy. The classic example of this is relationship between smoking tobacco and cancer. "In response to mounting evidence that smoking is harmful, the industry launched a campaign in the mid-twentieth century to stress that, despite what had been published in the scientific literature, the dangers of smoking had not been 'proven' and the results were little more than statistics. Any lack of consensus among researchers has therefore been [spun] by the tobacco industry in its continued insistence that even the experts 'don't really know' what makes smoking harmful."[45] Certain actors will take the uncertainty inherent in scientific studies and spin the issue to make it seem that the findings aren't as solid as they really might be. This has obvious consequences for political actors in the types of decisions that they may come to in regulating cancer-causing agents and sponsoring cancer research.

A less well-known example of the role of risk and uncertainty in cancer policy was the development of a means through which citizens living downwind of nuclear test sites might be compensated for instances of cancer that might be due to the nuclear fallout they experienced.[46] Because doctors could not with any certainty declare that any given case of cancer was due to radiation exposure, Congress ordered the National Institutes of Health to develop statistically based risk tables estimating the likelihood given the type of cancer and the amount of exposure the individual had that their cancer was due to the nuclear tests. Even these tables were heavily criticized because scientists could not agree on the appropriate methodology for applying risk. Add in political elements related to nuclear weapons, the amount of money the compensation would require, and public interest groups, and it was all but inevitable that the tables would fail to satisfy anybody involved.[47]

Scientific pluralism, or multiple interpretations of scientifically based evidence, reduces the power of consulting to the experts and doing as they say.[48] If even the experts can't come to some firm conclusion, why should we listen to them in the first place? The number of actors involved in giving meaning to scientific knowledge have only increased in recent years as they try to "contest and control scientific knowledge."[49] Social movements, interest groups, industry, doctors, and even patients themselves have become active players in interpreting and giving meaning to supposedly value-neutral facts. And the continued changing of the guard in regulatory agencies and politics as a whole virtually guarantees that priorities and interpretation of risk are constantly changing.[50]

Moving into the Political Arena

When the data and scientific opinion are unclear or uncertain, there is room for dissent. Different groups can take advantage of this dissent, even if it's slight. As a result, the discussion and debate over scientific research and findings can become political. An example of how uncertainty is often adjudicated by the political community comes in the Laetrile controversy of the 1960s and 1970s. Laetrile is a chemical related to vitamin B_{17}, which proponents claimed was at a deficit in cancer patients; if you were to provide Laetrile to cancer patients or proactively to those without cancer, the claim was that cancer could be vanquished.[51] While some animal evidence had been published and there existed case studies from Mexico on its supposed effectiveness, Laetrile was largely derided by cancer researchers. Despite this, cancer sufferers clamored for the drug, and many went to treatment centers in Mexico to be treated with it. In a profession dependent on peer review of research for advancement, the more mainstream scientists often prevented Laetrile studies from being published, and pro-Laetrile scientists moved to the fringe of the community.[52] This is but one example of how the process of peer review can discriminate and prohibit certain areas of study; in the case of Laetrile, the drug truly did not work, but it is not hard to imagine a case where another drug might truly work but be discriminated against by the main scientific community.

As a result of the public desire for Laetrile and the scientific community's unwillingness to recognize it and use it, "pro-Laetrile forces . . . expanded the conflict into the ideological, legislative and political arenas."[53] These proponents claimed that patients' access and ability to use Laetrile turned on freedom of choice, "that cancer patients have a right to choose their form of treatment without interference by the medical community or the government."[54] Pro-Laetrile scientists and patients were joined in their campaign by various interest groups who also supported this Libertarian-type ideology, like the John Birch Society and the Committee for Freedom of Choice in Cancer Therapy. These groups took their campaign to the courts, challenging the ban on the interstate sale of Laetrile. Today, Laetrile is still not approved by the FDA, and the NCI states that it has shown little effectiveness in fighting cancer. Although this is an example of controversy over an ineffective drug moving into the political arena, a more common controversy that tends to erupt is over the availability of drugs that appear to be effective in fighting disease, including cancer. This topic will be taken up in Chapter 3.

In entering the political arena, new principles are invoked, including ideological, judicial/administrative, and ideas about the role of government. Ideological disputes are involved in everything from ideas of freedom of choice, like the case of Laetrile, to ideas about the role of science in controversies like global warming. Unfortunately, the Republican Party in the United States has been connected with anti-intellectual and antiscience arguments.[55] This makes some of them predisposed to dislike or disagree with certain areas of scientific research and exploration (certainly this should not be taken to be a blanket statement, merely a statement that the tendency is present). Further, when science is made into a political controversy, the standards of decision-making are quite different. Instead of scientific consensus and peer review, government bodies focus far more heavily on the technical process of gathering evidence, analyzing it, and making decisions.[56] Because of laws such as the Administrative Procedures Act and the availability of the courts for adjudication of disputes, regulatory agencies are far more technical and transparent in making decisions, opening the door for other actors to get involved judicially. Regulatory agencies have become sensitive to the types of evidence that can be reliably used for making decisions.[57] This can lead to policy stalemate as different actors challenge the rulings in administrative and federal court. Finally, some conservatives would like to shrink the role of government, and in particular the regulatory agencies often involved in creating cancer policy. Why?

For most, they believe in smaller government and loosening the grip of regulations on business and industry; one need only look at the history of the Reagan administration and the minimization of the EPA for proof of this agenda. Implicit in this argument is the idea that it is not government's role to be involved in such broad areas; this reflects the Laetrile arguments that people should be free to choose their own treatment paths and options.

When government becomes the mediator for scientific disputes, the result is often that no one is happy. "Without the constraints of certain knowledge, the regulation of risk becomes intensely political."[58] Policy making and regulating for cancer are ultimately about how we deal with, understand, and mitigate risk. And unfortunately, there is no unanimously agreed on approach for doing this, especially when the science is unclear. The examples about estrogen replacement therapy and A/D discussed earlier are simply examples of how different governments understand risk differently and therefore decide differently about how to act. This has deeply affected cancer policy and therefore the way we understand and treat cancer.

Can Government Responsibly Make Cancer Policy?

Given the difficulties that scientists have in coming to an agreement or consensus about important and relevant aspects of science, how could we ever expect government to be able to make science policy? Even if the science was unanimous, politicians would probably still disagree on how to interpret the uncertainty inherent in scientific findings. Where science is supposed to be value neutral, politics most certainly is not. You cannot divorce the politics from policy making; interpreting evidence and making decisions about what to do with it is a political act. Even regulatory bodies like the EPA, which are required to use the most advanced scientific data to support their decisions, are ideological and technical. For example, when the Republicans became the majority in both chambers of Congress in the 1994 elections, regulatory bodies severely curtailed their regulatory actions to better coincide with the political and ideological inclinations of their political masters.[59]

Another difficulty in supporting cancer research is the piecemeal budgeting regimen that happens on an annual basis. W.D. Kay argues with respect to the space program that the annual budgeting process shortchanges large-scale research and development projects that rely on consistent and long-term funding.[60] If a research project is undertaken in one year with the expectation of regular funding over a series of years, which is then reduced in the coming years, the scope of the project will also need to be cut back or project leaders will need to find additional sources of funding. Kay goes on to argue that democracies like the United States with such a budgeting process make carrying out large-scale science and technological projects, projects into which cancer research would fall, practically impossible.

There are other aspects of politics that make formulating cancer policy equally difficult. Cancer has often been tied to very political and controversial policy areas like health care reform, social security, and entitlements. In fact, some of the earliest presidential comments about cancer specifically referenced it in connection to these policy areas. This means that cancer is often drawn into constitutional issues of government ability to act and get involved in health care reminiscent of the recent judicial arguments over the constitutionality of the Affordable Care Act. And perhaps most disconcerting of all, the underlying motivations of groups that are interested in cancer policy might actually be to not solve cancer at all. To briefly preview the argument that will be discussed in Chapter 6, groups like the American Cancer Society or the pharmaceutical industry would stand to lose economically if cancer were all of a sudden cured. Even research into political behavior recognizes that politicians would prefer to appear to be solving a problem without ever solving it all, lest they lose an issue they could potentially campaign on.

In sum, both science and politics combine to make cancer policy a difficult topic for anyone to tackle. As numerous scholars have argued, science and scientific knowledge is a socially constructed animal dependent on societal norms and values for its direction and interpretation. Being value neutral in either cancer research or making cancer policy is practically impossible, and yet that is the task that government has taken upon itself. It is that task which this book will now turn to.

Cancer Policy in the United States: A Theory

Given this state of affairs, how can we explore the disparate regulatory, research, and scientific policy agendas pursued in the United States regarding cancer? The theory that will be pursued here is that U.S. cancer policy has emerged out of competition between political actors and institutions responding to political, social, scientific, and economic pressures of the type described earlier. Understanding how these factors affect political institutions and therefore how those institutions respond is critical to understanding the form and type of cancer policy that has emerged in the United States since the war on cancer began.

To more fully understand these interactions, this book will undertake an institutional analysis of the president, Congress, bureaucracies, and interest groups focusing specifically on the political, social, scientific, and economic pressures facing each as they attempt to shape cancer policy. The ultimate aim is to understand who the major players are and why they take the policy actions they have taken. Based on this analysis, I will argue that due to the confluence of these various pressures, the cancer policy that has been made in the United States has been piecemeal and insufficient despite repeated calls for a war or moonshot effort to cure cancer. The fact that the government cannot create such a comprehensive, cohesive policy means that the policy that has been instituted is inadequate and poor in making any sustained effort at curing cancer.

Even more than the government's inability to undertake a cohesive cancer policy, I will argue that even if they wanted to, a liberal democratic government of the type practiced in the United States is simply incapable of making the comprehensive type of policy needed to fully combat the cancer epidemic. The motivations to do so simply don't exist on the part of the cancer establishment, nor on the part of the politicians to support an all-out assault on cancer. This is on top of the pressures faced by each institution in creating and implementing cohesive policy.

This exploration will proceed as follows. In the next chapter I will undertake an examination of funding patterns for the National Cancer Institute, the main method through which the government funds cancer research. This quantitative analysis will show that funding for the NCI does not fall into any one category of budgeting theory such as incrementalism or distributive politics; rather, salience of cancer and defense spending are key influences on cancer spending. The budgetary analysis will be followed by a deeper look not only at the NCI but other bureaucratic agencies deeply involved in cancer policy like the EPA, National Institutes of Health, and the Food and Drug Administration.

Chapter 4 will examine the role and influence of the presidency in setting cancer policy. In addition to the Nixon declaration of war, other presidential initiatives and events have been equally important, including Ronald Reagan's cancer scare, Jimmy Carter's recent battles with melanoma, and President Barack Obama's recent call for a "moonshot" effort to cure cancer. Chapter 5 will look at congressional efforts on cancer policy, including a look at the ideological and partisan battle lines that often shape the making of cancer policy and influence congressional battles. Finally, Chapter 6 will focus on the rest of the cancer establishment, including medical professionals, research scientists, interest groups like the American Cancer Society, and the pharmaceutical industry. This chapter will also document how the insurance industry and Medicare and Medicaid influence cancer treatment and innovations.

None of this is too terribly hopeful for the millions of cancer patients and their families whose worst fears are in the process of being realized.

I do not and cannot believe that the people involved in setting cancer policy are cognizant of the underlying motivations influencing their actions or that they are purposefully making it difficult to find a cure for cancer. I am simply arguing that the institutions of the U.S. government make it difficult for well-meaning individuals to make significant inroads not only into cancer but other scientific areas. Perhaps in recognizing and understanding the patterns that are taking place in cancer policy, it will make it slightly easier for political actors to cross the aisle and come together on an issue that's very likely to touch every one of our lives.

CHAPTER TWO

Identifying the Culprits

The incidence of cancer is a sad side effect of modern living. With the conquering of curable or treatable diseases such as the plague, yellow fever, tuberculosis, or polio, people live longer and healthier lives than ever before. Unfortunately, living longer allows a greater time for our cells to turn against us and mutate into something that kills. Based on the latest statistics, one in two men and one in three women are at risk of developing cancer at some point in their lifetime; one in four men and one in five women will die from it.[1] Chances are that even if you are not personally afflicted with cancer, someone close to you will be. With such a growing prevalence of cancer in all parts of the body, treatment and research become central concerns. The vast majority of money dedicated to this task comes from the federal government; as of 2012, since the National Cancer Institute's (NCI's) inception in 1937, the U.S. government has devoted over $90 billion to cancer research.[2] In 2012 alone, the NCI was appropriated $5 billion, with private research dollars totaling $2.2 billion.[3] Unlike many other forms of scientific research with isolated teams working on projects independently of one another, cancer research, because of the multicenter experimental study approach, requires a coordinating body. That body is the NCI, thereby endowing it with a special importance and responsibility in the treatment of cancer. Despite presidential calls for a "war on cancer" dating to Richard Nixon and continuing on to Barack Obama's call for a "moon shot" style effort at curing it in his State of the Union in 2016, the American political establishment has seemingly thrown money at a problem whose solution has not become any clearer. The seeming failure of cancer research to find a cure (or cures) is in stark contrast to the pattern of increased funding for the NCI. A number of commentators have called the war on cancer a failure and a flop, and yet the funding continues.[4] Epstein goes so far as to blame the "cancer establishment" itself for misleading the American public into "believing that 'we are winning the war against cancer,' with 'victory' possible only given more time and money."[5] Is this seeming indifference to cancer funding actually a malignant process? What are the political contours of government funding of cancer research?

In the coming chapters, I will explore the individual political actors and institutions in more depth, but to get an overall look at the political, social, scientific, and economic factors involved in cancer policy, this chapter lays out in detail the variables that I will argue affect cancer policy generally and, more specifically, funding for cancer policy through the NCI. These variables include ideology, interest groups, saliency, distributive politics, and the economic health of the country, all of which will be used in later chapters to structure the institutional analyses of important actors in cancer policy.

Cancer Politics

In turning to a discussion of the types of political variables that might be involved in cancer funding, there has actually been a spectacular lack of attention paid to the topic on the part of political scientists. However, research on general science policy, along with budgeting theory, can help inform us as to the directions we should be looking in when it comes to cancer. For our purposes then, we can focus on these elements: political party and ideology, distributive (or pork barrel) politics, budgeting trade-offs and policy, policy proposals, and political crises.

Partisan Politics

It's hard to believe that something like cancer, which doesn't care about your party affiliation, could have a partisan tinge to it. And yet Proctor, in his book *Cancer Wars*, argues that politics itself has been an integral factor in cancer funding and prevention efforts.[6] His history suggests that ideologically influenced administrations, including those of the Carter and Reagan presidencies, had significant effects on cancer prevention and funding. Consistent with the overall regulatory cuts suffered under the Reagan administration, Proctor details how environmental prevention efforts in the form of Occupational Safety and Health Administration (OSHA) and Environmental Protection Agency (EPA) regulations were dramatically scaled back from Carter-era levels.

This work suggests that although politicians of all stripes may in principle support the idea of curing cancer or supporting cancer research, there are embedded issues in cancer policy that lend themselves to party politics. These elements include budgetary and regulatory politics, as well as general attitudes toward science policies. To begin with general attitudes toward science, again, it does not instantly strike many of us that supporting science would be a political football to be tossed about. And yet, Democrats and Republicans have strikingly different attitudes not only about science, but also about different types of science. For example, space policy, decisions about whether and when to send humans into outer space, has been shown to be a Republican issue.[7] Why would space be connected with Republicans? From the beginning of the space race in the late 1950s, spaceflight has been connected with military competition with the Soviet Union in the context of the Cold War; given Republican support for military issues, spaceflight tends to fall inside the greater realm of military policy.

Of late, there have also been trends within the Republican Party of less support for science funding in general. Although there hasn't been any substantial research into this trend, there are some suggestions as to its origin. One possible source is the evangelical element of the Republican Party. In many fundamental churches, members are taught to discount basic tenets of science such as evolution and the Big Bang theory for a greater reliance on the teachings of the Bible. These pastors preach that scientists are continually changing their minds and their beliefs, whereas the Bible presents concrete revelations of God's plans for the world. Some of these same churches also discount the value of higher education with its dominance by liberal professors, thus inculcating distaste, if not intense dislike, for elements of science and higher learning. Because the evangelical community has made up an increasing proportion of the Republican Party, it would only be natural for Republican politicians to adopt similar policy positions, discounting the role of and place for scientific research and development.

A further attitude that could contribute to the decline of Republican support for science is a growing libertarian dimension to Republican thought. This strain of ideology holds that government should be as small as possible, only involving itself in those areas where it absolutely must. The presidential campaigns of Ron Paul in 2008 and 2012 and by his son, Senator Rand Paul, in 2016 demonstrate this libertarian ideology. Senator Paul, along with other major Republican candidates, advocated reducing the scope of government and variously calling for the abolition of government agencies ranging from the Internal Revenue Service (IRS) to the Department of Education. Under this ideology, why should the government contribute to scientific development when it could reduce the scope of government? In reducing government, politicians could then cut the budget and then taxes.

Even for those Republicans who may not subscribe to libertarian or evangelical philosophies, many, if not the vast majority of, Republicans today support the overall reduction of the federal budget. The budgetary politics of the past several years reflect just how significant a policy position this has become. Republican desires to reduce the budget to reduce the deficit and debt have led to numerous budgetary stalemates and, in extreme cases, government shutdowns. Unfortunately, research and development has come in for a heavy hit in budgets along with other areas of government. Since 2006, government spending on research and development has fallen by 9.2 percent, or approximately $15 billion dollars.[8] Thus, even if politicians wanted to increase spending on cancer research, they will immediately run into the problem of finding the money to pay for it in incredibly difficult budgetary times.

Finally, regulatory politics, a key element of cancer policy, necessarily colors cancer in a partisan light. Numerous scholars have noted the Republican aversion to imparting an excessive number of regulations.[9] The classic example of this posture was the administration of Ronald Reagan, who came into office determined to alleviate the burden of what he saw as unnecessary regulations on industry. The Reagan ire for regulations fell particularly hard on the EPA for which Reagan nominated Anne Gorsuch to be the administrator. Under Gorsuch, the EPA came in for intense criticism, ultimately leading to the censure of Gorsuch by Congress. However, the Republican influence on regulatory politics has been felt elsewhere, for instance, with the 1994 Republican revolution, the George W. Bush administration, and the continued criticism by Republicans of what they see as excessive and illegal regulations put forward by the Obama administration. Because regulations form an essential and significant part of cancer policy, it is not hard to make the leap, then, that cancer, at least the regulatory element of it, is influenced by political party.

Pork Barrel Politics

One element of politics that tends to span the often large partisan divide is that in order to get power in politics, you must be elected by the voters. One of the ways in which elected officials have sought to do that is by bringing home the bacon—in other words, bringing government funds back to their district or state. Another way in which to view cancer research is through the lens of whether this policy area qualifies for the label of distributive or pork barrel politics. Weingast, Shepsle, and Johnsen define distributive politics as "those projects, programs, and grants that concentrate the benefits in geographically specific constituencies while spreading their costs across all constituencies through generalized taxation."[10] However, other scholars writing in this vein relate distributive politics to the idea of universalism: that "every district receives some amount of federal spending" so that every member of a legislature can sign on to the bill.[11] These ideas are obviously related in the sense that all legislators seem to want to bring home government money to their constituents, theoretically in order to aid their reelection efforts.[12] But the difference between the ideas of distributive politics and universalism is the extent to which benefits are allocated; for the Weingast, Shepsle, and Johnsen argument, resources are handed out in an unequal fashion, whereas the Stein and Bickers argument implies that benefits are given out more evenhandedly. Although not in the scope of the research presented here, this definitional disagreement could be causing the wide variance in scholarly findings on patterns of distributive politics noted by Stein and Bickers, among others.[13,14]

In a sort of retrospective piece published in 1994, Weingast, reflecting on the distributive politics literature up to that point, proposed four criteria for distributive policy, including:

(D1) Divisibility: Its projects are local and can be varied in size, scope, and dollar amount independently of one another.

(D2) Omnibus: It is an omnibus of many divisible projects within a policy area.

(D3) Expenditure: The legislation is an expenditure policy; its main task is to allocate a given amount of funds.

(D4) Scope: A large, supramajority of districts is eligible for funds.[15]

These criteria seem to incorporate the idea of universalism (that every district gets something) in that he specifies that a supramajority of districts is eligible. As such, and to avoid the equally sticky prospect of sorting through the conceptual debate, those criteria will be used here as a definition for distributive politics.

Although funding for the NCI may not seem to fit these criteria, when we look at how the NCI actually operates, another impression is formed. For 2013, the last year for which overall numbers are available, intramural funding (dollars put toward research done *by* scientists at the NCI) equaled $811.6 million dollars, whereas extramural funding (dollars given to outside scientists through grants, with the number of grants being 1,095) was more than double that at $2 billion dollars. The grants are distributed to cancer centers and research institutes across the United States, all of which benefit local communities through their findings or through economic benefits in attracting medical professionals. Previous research has shown that the presence of hospitals or research institutes does increase the amount of federal funds that states and districts receive.[16] Given this, it can be argued that cancer funding, although universal in its benefits, is pork barrel politics because of the way NCI funds cancer research; not only are projects divisible and omnibus, but the main purpose of the legislation is to appropriate money, and a large number of districts are eligible for the funding.

If we accept the premise that cancer research is distributive in nature, then the literature on pork barrel spending opens up a new line of inquiry into the politics of cancer. We might expect that cancer research may take on a nonpartisan bent with nearly all legislators voting in favor of cancer research and funding. This is incidentally supported by Smith[17] and Mintrom,[18] who argue that the presence of medical schools and/or research institutes in an area can lead to competitive forces for research grants. Because many medical schools and programs depend on a certain level of federal grant money, they often become entrepreneurial in nature, becoming specialized in certain areas and creating larger and larger affiliations of facilities.[19]

Whereas some have found empirical support for a universalistic/distributive expectation,[20] others have been critical of the hypothesis. Previous research has demonstrated that the behavior of legislators in seeking specialized funding of this sort is conditional on electoral vulnerability,[21] whereas others have found that political polarization and fragmentation of government can affect the extent of distributive politics.[22]

Budgeting Policy and Trade-offs

Another possible framework through which we could view cancer funding is incrementalism. This line of thought dates back to the 1950s and 1960s with work by Charles Lindblom and Aaron Wildavsky.[23] Incrementalism is the idea that an agency's or entity's budget in a given year is based on its budget in the previous year. The assumptions that underlie this theory include the idea that rational lawmakers limit their attention to a policy or agency in a given year by basing its next year's activities on what they had done previously, with few, if any, large jumps or changes in its activities. Berry summarizes the common conceptions that have come along with budgetary incrementalism, among them restricting the number of alternative, limited assessments of policy consequences, simple decision rules, and smallness of the ultimate change.[24]

The literature on incrementalism, like distributive politics, is wide, varied, and just as mixed; indeed, Berry argues that the idea of incrementalism, as expounded on by various scholars over the years, has become too varied and therefore no longer meaningful.[25] Despite this, the basic idea of incrementalism—that the budget in one year is based on the budget from the previous year—remains and could be powerful in explaining cancer spending.

One final way that we can examine the politics of cancer policy is a combination of partisan and budgetary politics. In the recent case of funding for the Zika virus, Republican politicians have been hesitant to vote for a large package of funds without either finding a way to fund it or taking the funds from elsewhere. This implies that funding for one area could come as a result of a trade-off from another area. Surprisingly, this is not a new approach to budgeting; one of the more comprehensive analyses examining this subject questioned whether there was a budgetary trade-off between defense spending and health spending. Peroff and Podolak-Warren, in an analysis spanning 1929–1974, found that there were some limited trade-offs in appropriation requests for health research during the years of the Korean War but none in other years.[26] Given the connections between military funding and cancer research noted in Chapter 1, this could be an interesting connection between budgetary policy, cancer research, and military funding.

Proposals and Crises

A common political saying is to never let a crisis go to waste. The saying is popular because public policy is easier to change when it has been shown to fail or go awry.[27] If presidents, or any policy entrepreneur for that matter, want to change or make their mark on any policy, crises are usually the time to do it. There are clear examples where presidential policy pronouncements have affected cancer policy, with Nixon's war on cancer being the prime example. But what about other events, other proposals?

Focusing events are those events that are "sudden; relatively uncommon; can be reasonably defined as harmful or revealing the possibility of potentially greater future harms; has harms that are concentrated in a particular geographical area or community of interest; and that [are] known to policymakers and the public simultaneously."[28] The types of focusing events that we may encounter in terms of cancer would be instances where well-known individuals announce that they have or may have cancer, situations where publicized reports might focus attention on different aspects of cancer, or even large increases or decreases in cancer incidence and/or death. In the history of government attention to cancer, we can point to several instances where focusing events have occurred. The first one happened in the 1930s where increased media attention led to legislation establishing the NCI in 1937, and the second major one was clearly Mary Lasker, the American Cancer Society (ACS), and their push to make cancer a public health issue.

Ironically, two such focusing events occurred during the administration of Ronald Reagan, which, as previously noted, had been especially hostile to regulations that would have possibly led to fewer cases of cancer. First, in 1985, the president himself was subject to a colon cancer scare when a polyp was found during a routine colonoscopy. Because these types of polyps often turn out to be malignant, Reagan underwent surgery to remove it at which time doctors discovered a second polyp in his colon. When that polyp was removed a week later, it was indeed found to be malignant. With the tumor removed, doctors did not detect any further incidence of cancer, and the president was pronounced healthy. Despite this, the possibility that a sitting president might be diagnosed with cancer and undergo the treatment that is involved with such a diagnosis was a particularly startling one. Although plenty of presidents prior to Reagan suffered illness while president, demonstrating that being president and being ill could be done, Reagan served in a period in which media scrutiny was constantly increasing; the fact that he was the oldest serving president at the time made his health scares particularly an issue.

The very next year, Reagan's wife, Nancy, also underwent surgery for a malignant tumor in her breast. Although President Reagan's cancer case came in for far more scrutiny, the fact that within a year, the most well-known people in the United States, and perhaps the Western world, had themselves been afflicted by the disease brought greater attention to issues surrounding cancer in the United States. In 1985 alone, *The New York Times* published 95 stories on cancer compared with 70 in 1984 and 75 in 1986, demonstrating that far more attention was paid to cancer, most likely as a result of President Reagan's experience with it.

These examples all indicate the power that focusing events and policy proposals can have not only on public policy in general, but specifically cancer policy. These types of focusing events have the effect of turning public and political attention to issues that may have fallen off the policy agenda and putting greater pressure on the political establishment to do something, anything, to alleviate them.

The Social Side of Cancer

Occurrences of Cancer and Public Saliency

One of the most direct ways in which we come to know about cancer is when it affects either ourselves or someone close to us. When that happens, our knowledge about the scourge of cancer and its impact becomes immediately clear and we become invested in seeing a solution found. The original impetus for the founding of the NCI in 1937 was a sharp increase in cancer occurrences, which led to increased public awareness.[29] One way, then, that we can examine influences on cancer policy is through incidences of cancer and public awareness of a problem, something that scholars have recognized as an important element of the policy process.[30]

From 1975, the first year for which we have reliable data, to 1992, incidences of all types of cancer increased from 400.4 cases per 100,000 individuals to 510.7 cases per 100,000. Following this peak, incidences of cancer leveled off somewhat and began to decline consistently in 2007. Clearly then, for most of this history, citizens were beginning to have a far more personal experience with cancer, something that could easily contribute to increased attention to cancer and public support for cancer research.

One way to gauge public interest in cancer is to utilize public opinion poll results, but there is no poll that consistently asks about the importance of cancer to an individual. In the following analysis, I use the number of *New York Times* articles on cancer to gauge saliency, but there is a newer method that can shed light on public interest, at least since 2004: Google searches. Google Trends offers a glimpse at the rate at which people search for various terms, in this case, cancer. They report search frequency on a scale of 1 to 100, with 100 being the highest frequency of searches in the given time period, with searches then scaled to that for the rest of the period. Figure 2.1 provides this information for January 2004 through May 2016. The first thing to notice is that searches about "cancer" tend to

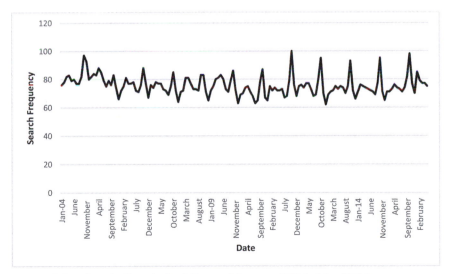

Figure 2.1   Google Trends for "Cancer," January 2004–May 2016

be relatively consistent and consistently high. The second pattern of note is that there are yearly spikes in searches during the month of October. Why October? October happens to coincide with Breast Cancer Awareness Month, with its large number of events from road races to screenings and which is often celebrated by a burst of pink from Washington, D.C., to the football fields of the National Football League (NFL). In fact, the search data peak in October 2011. These peaks in the months of October are significant; they demonstrate the ability of concerted public awareness campaigns to move the dial on the level of public awareness. Although we would certainly like to see cancer awareness remain high year round, it demonstrates the power of interest groups which are discussed later.

Class Differences

Although it might not immediately appear that there might be a class element to cancer, if we think a little more about the causes of cancer, it becomes more plausible that socioeconomic status may play a role, if not in cancer cases then in the treatment of it. This connection between class and cancer has yet to be explored fully or more in-depth, but there has been some previous suggestion that class may play a role in health care. Stork argues that at least with regard to the oil-rich states of the Middle East, class differences play a significant role in who can access quality health care.[31] To give a rough approximation of whether this might be the case or not, we can calculate the correlation between the number of people in poverty per state and the number of cancer cases per state. Utilizing the most recent data (2012), we get a value of 0.964 (the closer the value gets to 1, the more highly correlated the two variables are). Certainly a number of other variables are involved in this relationship, but the correlation demonstrates that there might indeed be some underlying connection between class and cancer.

Another reason to think that this link might exist is if we consider the environmental causes of cancer, like asbestos, tobacco smoke (both primary and secondhand), and various chemicals used in manufacturing and production, then those who are the least economically advantaged seem to be the most vulnerable to exposure. In their critique of the state of the cancer establishment, Epstein et al. note the failure of the NCI to investigate cancer clusters "in the vicinity of nuclear power plants, petrochemical industries, and Superfund hazardous waste sites—areas disproportionately and discriminatorily located in low-socioeconomic African-American and other ethnic communities."[32] White-collar workers who spend most of their day in clean office spaces would not be nearly as likely to be in situations where they might be exposed to such dangerous chemicals. Whereas others may contend that those office workers are killing themselves slowly by sitting all day, we can all agree that they are probably not as exposed to asbestos or formaldehyde as those at the lowest end of the income scale.

Finally, class differences may be heavily involved in screening and treatment. For those who can afford health insurance or work in jobs where insurance is provided, they have the resources of annual cancer screenings like Pap smears, colonoscopies, or prostate exams. Even with the passage of the Affordable Care Act, there are still those who cannot afford insurance, particularly those in the so-called Medicaid "gap," who make too much to qualify for Medicaid but too little to get subsidies on the health care exchanges. In these cases, patients will not be able to pursue recommended screenings, let alone expensive cancer treatments. Further, for those who are unfortunate enough to get cancer, the high costs of treatment, even with insurance, can be an insurmountable burden. Insurance plans may not cover the thousands of dollars that advanced cancer drugs cost and, depending on your network, you may not be able to access the best oncologists in the area. This would especially be the case for those individuals on Medicaid who would need to seek out cancer treatment.

Public Interest Groups

Interest groups have been by far a large driver in cancer policy since the mid-20th century. Mary Lasker's work with the ACS was responsible for much of the political and public attention that was paid toward cancer, which would eventually lead to Nixon's declaration of a war on cancer. The ACS has been the largest source of private funds for cancer research and continues to raise close to $1 billion on an annual basis for cancer research.[33] The ACS has local offices in many communities and flagship events like the Relay for Life that continue to publicize their efforts.

This does not mean that the ACS has not come in for serious criticism. Davis indicts the ACS for their own failures in pursuing adoption of lifesaving policies such as the Pap smear and anticigarette stances.[34] Davis argues that the leadership of the ACS, particularly during the 1950s and 1960s, had too close of ties with tobacco industries and the American Medical Association, which itself was against the broader use of Pap smears.

Other interest groups have been equally important in driving attention toward cancer. Maureen Hogan Casamayou argues in *The Politics of Breast Cancer* that the confluence of a powerful grassroots movement (the National Breast Cancer Coalition), media attention, and a lack of an opposition to increased funding and research helped drive an increased political awareness of breast cancer throughout the decade.[35] Aside from the ACS and the National Breast Cancer Coalition, there are a large number of public interest groups involved in cancer, from more well-known ones like Susan G. Komen (of the eponymous Race for the Cure events), Stand Up 2 Cancer, and the American Leukemia and Lymphoma Society, to groups that focus on specific types of cancer, like the Kidney Cancer Association, American Brain Tumor Association, and the American Lung Association. These groups pursue various activities from fundraisers, to awareness campaigns, to screening events, all of which can promote public awareness and support feeding back into public saliency as discussed earlier.

The Science of Cancer

If you ask someone on the street what they think is the biggest factor involved in cancer research and policy, they will probably say medicine or science. It's hard to think that something as personal and immediate as cancer would have anything but science involved in determining everything from research to treatment. But as I've laid out in Chapter 1 and up to now, there are clearly larger players involved. And yet, much of what those other players can and cannot do is still dependent on cancer science and medicine. So what do we mean when we say science is a variable that affects cancer research and funding? What about science are we referencing? For our purposes here, the two ideas we'll be focusing on are scientific uncertainty and the usage of scientific appeals.

Scientific Uncertainty

In Chapter 1 we discussed the idea of scientific pluralism, or the fact that rather than being a field of united ideas, different groups of researchers believe different facts and even interpret the same facts rather differently. When such uncertainty creeps into even the scientists, it's hard for that not to affect how politicians view and treat cancer policy. What happens when there are competing interpretations of scientific information? Not only is there confusion as to what the correct interpretation is, but "[t]he competition for the attention of peers, donors, editors, public officials, and customers is so intense that the irresistible temptation is to shout in order to be heard."[36]

One concrete example of how scientific uncertainty has played a role in cancer policy was at the end of the 1970s. Rushefsky argues that one of the stimuli for Reagan's regulatory retrenchment in the 1980s was the changing tide in cancer research at the end of the 1970s.[37] With more knowledge developing as to the mechanisms of carcinogenesis, the new scientific literature suggested that what government had been doing up to that point to regulate carcinogens was not effective. At the same time, multiple agencies and panels throughout the federal government were developing guidelines for how to consider and interpret the evidence about carcinogenic products and accompanying risk assessments. From the 1976 EPA guidelines to OSHA and the Interagency Regulatory Liaison Group, there was no one authoritative set of guidelines for assessing the risk offered by possible carcinogens.[38] This demonstrates just how slippery cancer policy was at the time, reflective of the uncertainty within the oncology field itself. However, as the state of the art advanced, newer information contributed to better knowledge and a better handle on the means by which we can mitigate cancer risks. We can expect, then, that as the field of cancer medicine expands, we might be able to make more effective policy, knowing exactly what causes cells to turn against their hosts.

Utilization of Scientific Arguments

When politicians think about the types of appeals they are going to make about something, such as why they should be elected by their voters, they can select from a wide variety of things to aid them in making their argument. Emotional appeals, rational appeals, psychological appeals, even economic appeals—politicians can reach us through our hearts, minds, or even our pocket books. Often, they find that emotional appeals tend to be the most effective; it's what drives us to protect our country in the military or stake out positions on issues that are nearest and dearest to us. Scientifically based appeals can also be used to support calls to arms; however, they may be less effective than some other types of rhetorical language. In a study of the usage of different types of appeals in regulating second-hand smoke, Lisa Bero and colleagues found that scientific appeals were less likely to appear in regulatory hearings, even though regulatory policy specifically calls for the consideration of scientific evidence.[39] Thus, even in the arena probably best suited for scientific evidence and arguments to be mustered, ideological, political, and economic arguments were still more likely to be cited.

In general, why might scientific appeals tend to fall flat compared with others? A first possible reason is the low level of scientific literacy in the United States. According to a 2015 Pew Research Center study, the ability of Americans to correctly answer basic scientific knowledge questions ranged from 86 percent (what is the Earth's hottest layer) to 34 percent (the temperature water boils at in high altitudes). This demonstrates that American scientific knowledge is probably not as great as it should be; if the American public cannot understand basic scientific facts, then they will probably not be able to understand the complicated means through which hypotheses are tested and conclusions are made. For example, a study published in 2016 about the effect of cell phone radiation on rats found that rats exposed to the type of radiation emitted from cell phones were more likely to develop tumors in the brain and heart. However, the study was performed on rats (which, as we've previously discussed, cannot be directly translated into conclusions about humans); furthermore, female rats exposed to the radiation did not develop the types of tumors that male rats did. The results of the study are clearly nuanced, but when people are subjected to headlines such as "New Study Raises Concerns of Possible Cell Phone Cancer Link" and cannot understand the details behind it, they are likely going to think twice about putting that cell phone to an ear (at least for five minutes).

The success of scientific appeals may also be diminished precisely because of the highly technical nature they entail. For the vast majority of the public, numbers are meaningless and boring. Knowing someone or having personally been affected by cancer is a far greater stimulator to action than being told that one out of three women or one out of two men are likely to have cancer in their lifetimes. Those faceless statistics often lead to the conclusion that that will never be me or my family; certainly I could never be affected. This depersonalization through numbers and science leads us to discount the scientific appeals.

Finally, scientific appeals are weakened when scientists, upon receiving new information, are forced to change their conclusions and arguments. Although this is only a natural part of the scientific process, it can be disconcerting when scientists must return to regulatory bodies and change their findings based on new information. This can particularly confuse the public who may be bombarded with conflicting information, as in the case of the cell phone–cancer link noted earlier. The headlines may inundate individuals with claims that cell phones cause cancer, but a new study months later could only add confusion and uncertainty to individual beliefs. They may come to believe that if science is so finicky, how can we believe anything the scientists have to say? If the public cannot understand the scientific process in the first place, they are likely to become even more confused and frustrated with shaky claims supposedly undergirded by science.

Even though science is the underlying mechanism by which regulatory agencies and politicians must make their decisions on cancer policy, the use of scientific appeals may actually weaken their ability to successfully make good policy. This appears as something of a catch-22; politicians need the data, but they cannot talk about it in a scientific way. This is particularly the case if the study methodology is suspect or able to be critiqued; by relying on scientific appeals, politicians open themselves up to possible criticisms and objections from those who disagree. Therefore, when we look at how scientific factors affect cancer policy in the United States and the actions made by different institutions, it is important to keep in mind the limiting factors of scientific appeals and arguments based on scientific fact.

The Economics of Cancer

Industry Interest Groups

The consideration of industry interest groups could fall under either politics or economics; I have decided to consider it under the heading of economics because at the end of the day, industry interest groups have a vested interest in protecting their own economic health. Industry interest groups are decidedly different from public interest groups; industry groups represent those organizations and individuals that are directly involved in and profiting from cancer research, treatment, and even the carcinogens themselves. Some of the most poignant attention to industry groups has come, naturally, in the form of criticism. Samuel Epstein's 1998 book, *The Politics of Cancer Revisited*, follows up on his original 1978 study, which, among other things, highlights the influence of industry on the influential National Cancer Advisory Board.[40] Meanwhile, Proctor details the confluence of science and public relations in describing how trade groups such as the Tobacco Institute and the Chemical Manufacturers Association have utilized the seemingly objective smoke screen of scientific knowledge to defend known cancer-causing agents, including tobacco, pesticides, and asbestos.[41] Both Epstein and Proctor argue that the involvement of business and trade groups have severely hampered government efforts at funding prevention and mitigation efforts.

In what is called the "classic exposé on the cancer establishment," Moss explicitly makes the argument that cancer is a big business.[42] From the doctors providing basic care to the specialists in radiology, oncology, radiation therapy, and palliative care, to the pharmaceutical industry who have recently faced criticism for skyrocketing drug costs, fighting cancer is a big industry.[43] The NCI has estimated that by 2020, the annual economic cost of fighting cancer will be *at least* $158 billion.[44] Given the costs involved, it is no wonder that some industries have an entrenched interest in seeing government investment in cancer care increase. In fact, some authors have gone so far as to speculate that the cancer industry does not mind "losing" the war on cancer[45]; as long as there is a war to be fought, they believe, the government will continue to fund their work.

The State of the Economy and the U.S. Budget

When looking at the federal budget in the United States, there are usually three large categories of spending: defense spending, mandatory expenditures (this includes entitlement spending and other spending required by law), and discretionary expenditures. In 2012 the discretionary portion of the budget made up only about 18 percent of the overall budget, and that part must include most of the things we ask government to do: education spending, transportation and infrastructure, veterans' affairs, diplomatic activities, and yes, scientific research and development. Because science spending ends up in the part of the budget that is discretionary, it is a part of those programs that are likely to see the budget axe when it comes time to balance the budget or reduce federal spending. A related issue is that as overall medical costs increase, the federal government is increasingly on the hook for rising Medicaid and Medicare costs. Both of these programs fall under mandatory spending, so because the federal government must devote more money to the mandatory areas, there are fewer funds to spend in discretionary areas.

Funds for scientific development are highly sensitive to the overall conditions surrounding the U.S. economy, which influence annual budgeting. When economic times are good and tax money is being added to the federal coffers, it is easy to decide to spend it in areas like research and development; a rising tide floats all ships. However, in poor economic times, discretionary items are usually the first to be cut. One example where we see this play out in science policy is with National Aeronautics and Space Administration (NASA) and the human spaceflight program. Conley and Whitman Cobb demonstrate that one of the biggest determining factors when Congress considered presidential requests for NASA was the overall U.S. economy; budgets rose when times were good and fell when they were bad.[46] In fact, funding for NASA began to fall dramatically in the mid-1960s *before* the United States ever reached the moon. Why? The increasing cost of the war in Vietnam, as well as Lyndon B. Johnson's Great Society programs, monopolized government money and attention. Other research and development projects have been cancelled or halted due to an increased budgetary need, like the previously mentioned Superconducting Super Collider.

In sum, we might expect to see funding for cancer research and policy increase when economic conditions make it easier for the government to spend more money. However, in periods where funds could be circumscribed, such as bad economic times or in periods where crises elsewhere in the world are consuming our attention and funds, it is easy to see how something like cancer could be shorted in favor of more essential government programs.

Methodology

Because no analysis of cancer funding has been performed before, it's only natural to ask how cancer funding fits into other conceptions of governmental funding. Does it accord with the patterns of science or health policy? Unlike much scientific research, however, cancer research is perhaps the area that touches a majority people, if not directly, at least very closely. Because of that, does it fit a more distributive pattern or follow electoral imperatives? Or is cancer funding a unique policy area following its own imperatives? Given this and the fact that government money has funded the vast majority of cancer-related research, it is surprising that there has been a lack of focus on this topic.

In order to uncover some of the drivers of cancer funding, two possible analyses could be conducted. The first, which will be performed later, involves a quantitative analysis of the NCI budget. This will allow us to establish a long-term broad overview testing some of the variables noted previously. A second, more specific analysis could also be done looking at a congressional vote on a cancer-related bill. In an analysis of this sort, we could look at more regional and local factors in predicting support for cancer funding, as well as other individual-level variables such as party and personal experience with cancer. Unfortunately, a number of obstacles prevent that sort of analysis. First, the budget for the NCI in recent years has not been voted on in a stand-alone appropriations bill; rather, it has been rolled in with other agencies or in a consolidated omnibus fashion. Second, recent cancer-related bills that have passed and become law are very few— the last time this occurred was 2008 when the Caroline Pryce Walker Conquer Childhood Cancer Act of 2008 and the Breast Cancer and Environmental Research Act of 2008 were passed. These two would be good candidates for such an analysis but for one major reason: the Conquer Childhood Cancer Act was passed by unanimous consent in the Senate and in a vote of 416–0 in the House, and the Breast Cancer and Environmental Research Act was also passed by unanimous consent in the Senate and a voice vote in the House.[47] As such, neither bill is appropriate to use here.

Excluding bills that have become law, we could find a resolution or bill that has been passed by one chamber and not the other. Examples of these abound, such as resolutions declaring National Prostate Cancer Awareness Month or the Recalcitrant Cancer Research Act of 2012; however, these types of resolutions and bills have all been passed via unanimous consent in the Senate or by voice vote in the House. A final reason an individual-level analysis is not performed here is that aside from these two bills, there are no other recent bills (by recent meaning since 2000) that could be considered. Performing the analysis in an earlier period of time would give no clue as to the dynamics of cancer funding today. What this does tell us, however, is that when the Congress does vote on cancer-related issues, members are generally supportive, seeing little controversy or cause to vote against such items.

Given the limitations noted earlier, I will only undertake the long-term budgetary analysis for the time period of 1975–2011. Although the NCI has existed since 1937, reliable statistics regarding cancer occurrence and death, which are included as major independent variables, are only available since 1972 and updated through 2011. As displayed in Figure 2.2, the NCI budget has risen fairly consistently from 1968 until 1999 when the budget was $292 billion. In 2000 this rose to $333 billion and in 2001 to $375 billion. Since then, the budget has remained remarkably stable, with 2014's budget number at $492 billion.

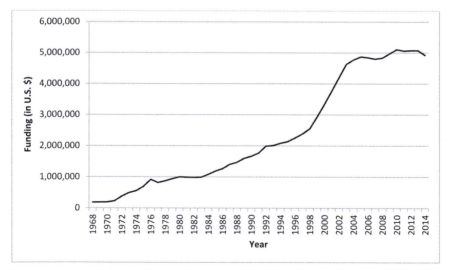

Figure 2.2 National Cancer Institute Funding (in millions), 1968–2014 (National Cancer Institute)

In simply examining Figure 2.2, the NCI budget appears to be incremental in nature for most of the series; this observation would fall in line with the incrementalism paradigm discussed earlier. This is rather astounding given that for most of this period, the politics of cancer were driven by Nixon's declaration of war against the malady in 1971 and Reagan's cancer scare in 1985, both of which would credibly be expected to increase funding for cancer research but appear not to have had any significant effect. Further, the rather quick jump in funding at the turn of the 21st century belies the traditional expectations of incrementalism with cancer funding leveling off afterward. Therefore, although incrementalism might appear to fit with the pattern of cancer funding, it does not account for the whole history of the series.

The next step in the analysis is to perform a quantitative analysis utilizing ordinary least squares (OLS). The NCI budget will be used as the dependent variable with independent variables to include the following:

Cancer Statistics. Utilizing data gathering by the NCI's Surveillance, Epidemiology, and End Results Program (SEER), the following cancer statistics will be used: annual cancer deaths per capita, number of new cancer cases per capita, and the cancer incidence rate per capita. All of these figures are available for 1972–2011.

Hospitals. Given Smith's research into health policy and its relation to the number of medical schools and research institutes in a given district,[48] a variable measuring the number of hospitals in the United States is included. Although this isn't directly reflective of the medical school/research institute argument, it does account for system capacity for caring for society's ill. This number is not available for every year, but is based on a census of U.S. facilities performed by the Centers for Disease Control (CDC) done on an average of every five years.

Budgetary Figures. Accounting for the findings of Peroff and Podolak-Warren,[49] I will include annual defense spending as a means of control (in billions of dollars). Additionally, the overall U.S. budget annually will be included.

Economic Variables. To control for changes in the U.S. economy that could potentially affect overall budgeting politics, I will include the annual U.S. gross domestic product (GDP) in the analysis.

Political Variables. In any policy area, there exists the chance for partisanship, or at least political ideology, to play a role. For example, if Republicans wish to shrink the size of government and decrease the budget, any funding increases, even if it is for an issue like cancer, may not be supported. In order to test for partisanship in cancer spending, I will include three political measures: the party of the president (measured as a dummy variable, 1 for Democrat), the number of Democrats in the House of Representatives, and the number of

Democrats in the Senate.[50] A variable indicating whether the year is an election year (congressional) is also included to account for possible increased spending in a pattern that would conform to the hypotheses of distributive spending.

Salience of Cancer. Because public awareness has been shown to play a role in a number of policy areas, I will include a measure for public salience of cancer. Perhaps the easiest way to measure such a thing would be public opinion surveys asking about public concern with cancer. However, because this question is not asked on a regular basis, I will be using an alternative means—the number of articles in *The New York Times* specifically about cancer. This number will include not only articles about politics and cancer, but also about cancer research and cancer awareness. As the "paper of record," *The New York Times* serves as a measure of what the public is interested in and aware of at any given time.[51] Additionally, I will include a dummy variable accounting for President Ronald Reagan's colon cancer scare in 1985 to account for increased public attention to the issue.

Gini Index. Finally, Stork has suggested that perhaps class differences play a role in medical research and funding, with the disproportionate benefit going to upper- and lower-class individuals, not the middle class.[52] In order to account for this, I will include the Gini coefficient for the United States each year.

Findings

Table 2.1 presents the results of three OLS models. Model 1 is a basic model incorporating all of the variables detailed earlier with NCI budget as the dependent variable. Although the model performs well, only one of the variables is significant: death rate per 100,000. However, the residuals of the model are heteroscedastic; as such, model 2 presents a second option, removing GDP from the independent variables (because it provided nothing to model 1) and logging the budget variables (NCI budget, U.S. budget, and defense spending) to account for the heteroscedasticity. A final model, number 3, is included as a means of testing for incrementalism. Model 3 lags behind the dependent variable, NCI's budget, by a year. According to the theory of incrementalism, the budget for year T would be dependent on the budget in year $T-1$.

In comparing the performance of the three models, they all explain the dependent variable fairly well with adjusted R^2 of 0.991, 0.995, and 0.990, respectively. This means that each model explains approximately 99 percent of the variation in the dependent variables. Because model 1 exhibits heteroscedasticity, the question is which model, 2 or 3, performs the best. Being slightly more efficient, model 2 is the best performer of the three.

Table 2.1 Regression Results

Variables	Model 1	Model 2 (Logged Budget Variables)	Model 3 (Logged Budget Variables; NCI Budget Lag)
Constant	11246639.86 (4868856.603)	78.416(0.503)***	8.800 (0.514)***
Death Rate per 100,000	−49585.565 (13427.503)***	−0.006 (0.001)***	−0.007 (0.002)***
Incidence Rate per 100,000	6360.477 (5229.407)	0.002 (0.001)**	0.003 (0.001)***
Defense Spending	3.399 (1.287)	0.302 (0.081)***	0.332 (0.107)**
GDP	0.000 (0.003)	—	—
Number of Democrats in House	−2214.692 (3538.440)	−0.001 (0.000)*	−0.001 (0.000)*
Number of Democrats in Senate	15855.128 (12232.213)	0.004 (0.002)*	0.003 (0.002)
Democrat as President	−298894.328 (114724.126)	−0.041 (0.013)***	−0.041 (0.016)**
Salience	3750.402 (3488.826)	0.001 (0.000)***	0.000 (0.000)
Reagan Scare	−67351.611 (225395.280)	−0.025 (0.030)	−0.040 (0.032)
Gini	11647503.34 (9756386.858)	1.039 (1.119)	1.549 (1.249)
U.S. Budget	−0.632 (0.345)	−0.021 (0.047)	−0.139 (0.053)*
Hospitals	−1164.084 (340.815)**	0.000 (0.000)	0.000 (0.000)*
Election Year	−9342.492 (68701.589)	−0.002 (0.009)	−0.008 (0.010)
	$R^2 = 0.991$	$R^2 = 0.997$	$R^2 = 0.994$
	Adj. $R^2 = 0.985$	Adj. $R^2 = 0.995$	Adj. $R^2 = 0.990$

***<0.001; **<0.01; *<0.05

So what do these results tell us about the political contours of cancer funding? Interestingly, the coefficient for death rate is counterintuitive; the sign is negative, meaning that as the death rate increases, the NCI budget falls. However, the coefficient is relatively small, indicating that perhaps this could be a spurious finding, particularly since the incidence rate coefficient is in the expected direction.

Defense spending is also found to be significant, but again in a direction not predicted by the literature. It seems that the United States does not make a trade-off between health and arms; as defense spending rises, so does the NCI budget. In fact, military spending appears intimately tied to cancer research; Casamayou notes that for breast cancer in particular, the military and, more specifically, the Department of the Army became an important source of money for research after money was specifically appropriated to them for the purposes of breast cancer research.[53]

Another interesting finding in this data is the role of political party. As the number of Democrats in the House rises, the NCI budget appears to fall, whereas the reverse is true of Democrats in the Senate. However, the trump card is often held by the president, and the model implies that when Democrats are presidents, the NCI budget falls. Therefore, given this combination of findings, Democrats, often lauded and criticized for their use of government funds (depending on perspective), seem to cut NCI funding, making cancer more of a Republican issue.

Salience, as measured by articles in *The New York Times*, is also highly significant, indicating that as public awareness of and interest in cancer rise, funding does as well. In model 2, Reagan's cancer scare, Gini, the U.S. budget, the number of hospitals, and election year are all insignificant.

Given the dearth of research into this topic and thus the uncertainty that necessarily creeps in as to which variables would be the most important, an additional statistical method could be of use. A stepwise linear regression takes a number of independent variable and through a series of statistical tests reports back which combination of variables might give us the most leverage over the data. Table 2.2 presents the stepwise regression results given the same model parameters as previously used.

The variables that the stepwise regression indicates are most important are defense spending, hospitals (both significant in all three models), salience, and Gini (significant in two out of three). These findings are somewhat different from those in Table 2.1 where both Gini and the number of hospitals are not significant. However, in models 2 and 3 of the stepwise regression, the number of hospitals is so tiny (it computes out farther than three decimal places) that its effect appears to be negligible. Given these findings, and combined with the results from the first round of regression analyses,

Table 2.2 Stepwise Regression Results

Variables	Model 1	Model 2 (Logged Budget Variables)	Model 3 (Logged Budget Variables, NCI Budget Lag)
Constant	943972.418 (3182579.863)*	8.696 (0.480)***	8.294 (0.519)***
Death Rate per 100,000	−33439.612 (5983.135)***	—	—
Incidence Rate per 100,000	—	—	—
Defense Spending	2.079 (0.599)***	0.487 (0.057)***	0.438 (0.074)***
GDP	—	—	—
Number of Democrats in House	—	—	—
Number of Democrats in Senate	—	—	0.003 (0.001)*
Salience	6622.612 (2324.739)**	0.001 (0.000)***	—
Reagan Scare	—	—	—
Gini	12844662.46 (5429443.095)*	—	3.208 (0.817)***
U.S. Budget	—	—	−0.156 (0.061)**
Hospitals	−1086.208 (262.542)***	0.000 (0.000)***	0.000 (0.000)***
Election Year	—	—	—
	$R^2 = 0.988$ Adj. $R^2 = 0.985$	$R^2 = 0.985$ Adj. $R^2 = 0.984$	$R^2 = 0.987$ Adj. $R^2 = 0.984$

***<0.001; **<0.01; *<0.05

it appears that salience and defense spending are the variables with the largest impact on NCI funding, followed by political party and death and incidence rates.

Analysis and Conclusions

This chapter began by asking whether governmental cancer funding (measured through the NCI budget) is most in line with the budgetary dynamics of health and science policy, distributive politics, or incremental-ism or is a category all of its own. The findings here suggest that the variables that influence the NCI's budget the most are not incidence or death rates, as one might suppose, but somewhat atypical from expectations. Beginning with the expectations of incrementalism, if this theory were to explain the NCI budget, we would expect that model 3, the lagged bud-getary model, would be best at explaining NCI budget patterns. It is true that model 3 in both the regression and stepwise regression performs excep-tionally, but it does not perform as well as the nonlagged models. This coincides with the pattern in funding noted earlier that although incre-mentalism appears to account for most of the NCI budget levels, it does not explain the significant increase and leveling off in the past 15 years.

Turning to the distributive politics framework, if this hypothesis is to hold true, political party should have no effect and the number of hospitals and election year would be significant. The first set of regressions does sug-gest that political party is significant; however, the findings are mixed and, although significant, are not as strong as some of the other variables. For hospitals, the findings are interesting. In model 3 in Table 2.1 and all three models in Table 2.2, the number of hospitals is significant; however, in three out of four models, the variable is significant, whereas the coefficient is 0 to three decimal places. The number of hospitals is only important to a minor degree, with election year not significant in any model. Thus, whereas the characteristics of cancer funding would suggest a distributive politics model to be best at describing funding patterns, this analysis would not concur. As noted earlier, an individual-level analysis of congressional roll-call voting would be helpful in exploring this further, but there are no avail-able data at this time.

The partisan aspect of the models is particularly intriguing because it suggests that Republicans are more supportive of funding for the NCI despite Republican qualms with increased discretionary and scientific funding. Although initially, a hypothesis about which party would better support cancer funding might turn on the Democratic Party, Republican presidents, in concert with Republican- led Senates, appear to increase funding more. Perhaps Republicans are more supportive of *funding* for cancer research than they are for regulations that might reduce the number of cancer cases altogether, a topic that will be taken up in the next chapter. However, an additional explanation for this finding might be that some sort of interaction is happening between party and defense spending. Both models also suggest a strong positive correlation between defense spending and NCI spending; because Republicans are generally more supportive of military and defense spending, these findings may indicate a complex relationship between military and health spending that are both related to partisan identification. As I've previously detailed, there is a significant relationship between defense research and spending and health research and spending; particularly with the advent of nuclear weaponry, the Department of Defense began to invest more heavily in health research. Those patterns continue today as the DOD struggles to understand the science behind things such as Gulf War syndrome, traumatic brain injuries, and mental illnesses like post-traumatic stress disorder (PTSD). Perhaps increased defense spending indicates increased military conflict; with increased conflict comes a heightened attention on the health and safety of troops, leading to increased focus on medical research, an aspect of which may bring the NCI into play.

The finding in Table 2.2 that Gini, the inequality index, is significant is interesting indeed. It would suggest that as economic inequality rises, so does cancer funding. This is interesting in that cancer is something that fundamentally affects everyone: rich, poor, employed, unemployed, Democrat, and Republican. The potential for this finding is mentioned only obliquely by Joe Stork in his 1989 "Political Aspects of Health." He argues that "[t]he health care strategies of any society have a significant class dimension: will resources be used primarily to improve nutrition, sanitation, and workplace environments, and the health of the base of the population, or to acquire expensive technologies that will benefit mainly those holding economic power."[54] However, again in light of the findings about party, the fact that more inequality leads to more funding for the NCI is something of an anomaly. If Republicans want to decrease funding for welfare and other means-tested social programs, we would not expect NCI funding to increase.

In sum, it appears that cancer funding is a unique area befitting its unique status as perhaps the only malady that affects all of us and therefore connects all of us. As such, it's pivotal that the government be involved in such an endeavor; but it's also appropriate that we ask what motivations lie behind the funding behavior, if not for ourselves, then for the people we know likely to be affected around us. These topics will be taken up in greater detail in the next several chapters. The in-depth evaluation that the next chapters offer will allow greater light to be shed on such a dark issue.

CHAPTER THREE

Bureaucracies and Cancer

On a recent Saturday evening, my husband and I were invited to go to the local midget car races. We went and shortly after we arrived at the track and found some seats, the smell of cigarette smoke reached me. Immediately, alarm bells of "Cancer! Cancer! Cancer!" went off in my head, most likely because I was in the middle of preparing this book. The negative health effects of secondhand smoke ran through my mind: not just cancer, but asthma, ear infections, chronic obstructive pulmonary disease (COPD). In fact, the Centers for Disease Control (CDC) on its website clearly says, "There is no risk-free level of exposure to secondhand smoke." I wondered where the smoking section was and I could find none. I struggled for breaths in between the wafts of smoke. Recognizing the danger from secondhand smoke, state and local governments throughout the country have slowly allowed for smoking bans in public places, or at least designated areas in which smokers can have their cigarettes, but that had clearly not worked its way down to the local race track. Where was the government protecting my rights to not have to be subjected to the health dangers of second-hand smoke? Taking it one step further, knowing and acknowledging the immense health costs of smoking to begin with (something even Nazi Germany recognized), why hasn't the government simply banned tobacco altogether? They've banned drugs such as marijuana, why not tobacco as well?

Let's take another example, one that has reached outside of the cancer community. In the late 1980s as HIV/AIDS was ravaging gay populations in America, drugs meant to control the infection were only just being inves-tigated. The drug AZT showed promise in early trials but before the Food and Drug Administration (FDA) had approved it, patients who were quickly dying were begging to be given the drug. The same was true of tamoxifen for breast cancer patients at around the same time. In fact, this is happening all the time. People dying of difficult diseases watch promising new drugs being tested and want to be given the opportunity to try to extend their lives by just a little bit more. This "right to try" movement harkens to the idea that medical decisions, even if they are made on the basis of unknown or uncertain information, should be made by patients in concert with their doctor. Why should some government organization have to give permission for any drug to be used? Why deny somebody the means by which they could extend their lives?

Both of these stories, however, can also be flipped around. What about the rights of those who smoke to be able to continue to do so? If we are going to give dying patients the right to decide what to do with their bodies, why shouldn't we give that to smokers? Knowing the health risks, if they want to continue to smoke, shouldn't they be allowed to? And what about the rights of the drug companies manufacturing potentially lifesaving drugs? If they give a trial drug to someone outside of a drug trial and it fails, it could potentially bring the entire trial to a halt. At the heart of both of these examples is the idea of rights, that we have the right to do as we wish with little or no interference from the government.

The language of rights is far more familiar in politics than it is in something like cancer. And yet, an individual's rights are what is at stake when government and their representatives get involved in activities such as research and development, making regulations, and approving new drugs. So where do one person's rights end and another's begin? How do you balance my right to not be subjected to secondhand smoke and the smoker's right to have a cigarette? How do you balance an individual's right to make their own medical decisions with the greater good of ensuring the safety of drugs in the country? The difficult task is not left so much with our elected officials but with the government bureaucracies and bureaucrats who are charged with carrying out laws and making these difficult choices.

This chapter will examine three bureaucracies in particular that are major players in cancer policy: the National Cancer Institute, the Food and Drug Administration, and the Environmental Protection Agency. Taken together, they are the three agencies most responsible for cancer policy and protection in the United States, and the effects of their decisions are felt by all Americans at some time or another. After exploring each of these players in turn, I will then examine the output of these agencies in the form of regulations concerning the prevention of cancer from 1995–2015. This will allow for another test of the political, social, scientific, and economic factors that go into making cancer policy in the United States.

The National Cancer Institute

Originally created in 1937, the National Cancer Institute (NCI) is the largest provider of funds for cancer research in the United States. As it is constituted today, its research laboratories and cancer centers across America do everything from basic research into the mechanisms and nature of cancer to clinical trials to treatment and training of oncologists and physicians. In fiscal year 2014, over 40 percent of the NCI's budget was dedicated to extramural grants, in other words, the funding of research performed by scientists outside of the NCI.

Among the centers and divisions of the NCI, offices are dedicated to intramural research (research performed within the NCI), cancer epidemiology and genetics, cancer biology, cancer control, cancer prevention, and treatment and diagnosis. Other offices falling under the NCI director include the Center for Cancer Training, Center to Reduce Health Disparities, and the Coordinating Center for Clinical Trials. However, one of the biggest efforts for the NCI comprises the 69 designated comprehensive cancer centers devoted to bringing all elements of cancer research and treatment together under one roof. "A Comprehensive Cancer Center is designed to organize cancer care and research so as to optimize the delivery of ever-more-effective early diagnosis, therapy, and prevention."[1] Given that 95 percent of cancer patients do not have access to clinical trials,[2] the role of the NCI cancer centers is to provide a centralized location for researchers and doctors not only to treat cancer patients but to educate the community as to the latest emerging research and treatment opportunities available.

The Politics of the NCI

As we saw in the previous chapter, there are intriguing elements of partisan politics involved in funding the NCI. Presidents and politicians of both political stripes have called for and supported major cancer efforts, most prominently Richard Nixon but more recently President Barack Obama and Vice President Joe Biden. In the wake of the death of his son, Beau, from a particularly vicious form of brain cancer, Vice President Biden has taken the lead on expanding efforts at curing cancer, this time avoiding the language of war and using the rhetoric of a "moonshot" style effort. In any case, the NCI and its efforts should not be classified as overtly political; at the very least, there are some partisan elements at play but not in any broad, organized manner.

What does aid the NCI in gaining funds is the fact that those funds can be dispersed to different geographical entities, thus supporting the reelection efforts of particular members of Congress. With somewhere around $2.5 billion available in grants through the NCI, researchers and laboratories across the country can apply for the money and receive the benefits of government funding. However, the NCI grant process is a competitive, peer-reviewed procedure; researchers submit applications, which are then reviewed and scored by their peers on the NCI's various review boards. Thus, the opportunity for members of Congress to interfere and direct funds is somewhat circumscribed, but increasing the amount of funds available does give the NCI more money to give away, thereby increasing the odds that researchers in their state or district will be able to receive a piece of the pie.

Where politics can play a role with the NCI is in the combination of public awareness and public opinion, along with lobbying by interest groups and policy entrepreneurs. This is precisely the tack that Biden has taken with his moonshot campaign. Biden, using the public bully pulpit afforded to him by the stature of his office, has tried to increase public awareness of and public support for cancer research with the hope that increased public support will lead to increased funding. This "going public" campaign is nothing new, particularly at the presidential and vice presidential level.[3] As a policy entrepreneur, Biden is taking advantage of the increased public focus on cancer to push for a two-pronged effort: one, increase resources both public and private, and two, bring together different elements of the cancer community to gather and share more information.[4] Whether this push will be successful remains to be seen but with his time as vice president coming to a close, Biden will lose the public platform he has for his efforts.

The Social Side of the NCI

Even though the NCI is the largest funder of cancer research in the United States, there is relatively little public awareness about the agency and its role. This makes the job of the NCI even more difficult in promoting public awareness and providing education. Figure 3.1 shows the Google Trends data for both "National Cancer Institute" and "American Cancer Society" and has an intriguing pattern. Overall, there has been a long and consistent decrease in searches for both, but the NCI regularly gets fewer searches than the ACS. This demonstrates that interest in the NCI, with all of its tools and activities, is significantly less among the American public than their interest in the ACS, with far fewer resources available to them.

Why might there be less recognition for the work of the NCI compared to other cancer organizations? Quite simply, knowledge of the American

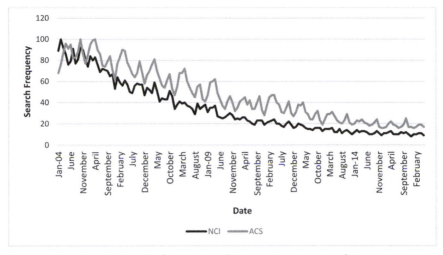

Figure 3.1 Google Trends for "National Cancer Institute" and "American Cancer Society," January 2004–May 2016

government in general is quite low; when you consider less well-publicized agencies like the National Institutes of Health and the NCI, it's only natural that public awareness would be low. Part of the problem may be on the part of the bureaucrats and the politicians themselves. In many of Vice President Biden's statements about the moonshot effort to cure cancer, the NCI is never mentioned; this is not an atypical situation. Despite the relative importance of the NCI to the fight against cancer, it is a rarely named player.

This lack of public awareness of the role of NCI means that it has relatively little political power compared to the ACS or other cancer actors. This could also contribute to the increasing cancer treatment disparities between socioeconomic classes. If the general public knows little about the NCI and its comprehensive cancer centers, it's easy to imagine that those in the worst economic positions know even less. This further adds to the lack of treatment opportunities and the availability of clinical trials that can impede cancer success overall.

The Science of the NCI

One area that has strongly influenced the operations of the NCI is the science of prevention and the NCI's attention, or lack thereof, to it. Because billions of dollars are available to researchers through NCI grants, NCI decisions as to what types of research to fund can have a significant impact on the direction that cancer research takes. In fact, some cancer researchers have taken specific aim at the NCI, arguing that the war on cancer is being lost and that the NCI lacks focus on prevention efforts.

Roughly 20 years after Nixon's declaration of war on cancer, many critics were alleging that the war was failing as cancer deaths and incidences continued to rise. As detailed in Samuel Epstein's *The Politics of Cancer Revisited*, Epstein, along with a number of other cancer researchers, argued beginning in 1992 that the NCI and the cancer establishment in general were at fault in the lack of progress made against cancer.[5] At the heart of the critique was the argument that

> . . . the NCI discounts the role of avoidable involuntary exposures to industrial carcinogens in air, water, food, the home, and the workplace. The NCI has also failed to provide any scientific guidance to Congress and regulatory agencies on fundamental principles of carcinogenesis and epidemiology, and on the critical needs to reduce avoidable exposures to environmental and occupational carcinogens. Analysis of the $2 billion NCI budget . . . reveals minimal allocations for research on primary cancer prevention, and for occupational cancer.[6]

Epstein and his colleagues argue that part of the reason the NCI discounts cancer prevention and environmental causes is that there are basic conflicts of interest within the NCI in connection with the pharmaceutical industry. This not only leads the NCI to primarily focus on profit-producing drugs, but to discount the extent to which environmental factors cause cancer.

This argument reflects the disputes within the scientific literature itself about the causes of cancer and therefore where scientific focus should reside. As the largest funder of cancer research, the NCI is a prime target for these critiques, and the situation has not changed dramatically since 1992. In 2013, only 6.2 percent of the NCI's budget was designated for prevention and control. However, to be fair, while the NCI certainly has the ability to research causes of cancer, they do not have the ability to enact regulations that would in fact *prevent* cancer; that job instead falls to regulatory agencies such as the EPA and Occupational Safety and Health Administration (OSHA). Indeed, while prevention is mentioned in the National Cancer Act of 1971 as an activity to be undertaken by the NCI and the National Cancer Program, it is not a main focus of the legislation. As such, for any major changes to come in the focus of the NCI, most likely major legislation would be called for to change the direction and attention of the NCI.

Despite these controversies, scientific developments are one area in which the NCI is not only influenced by but can actively influence in its disbursement of grants. The NCI issues several different types of grants, depending on the type of research being conducted and the amount of funds being requested. However, all competitive grants undergo a peer-review process. As previously discussed, peer review itself can be subject to significant bias and chance. Once a grant has been reviewed, the reviews along with the application are considered by the Scientific Program Leadership Committee, which considers not only the comments of the peer reviewers but "[c]ongressional mandates, new scientific opportunities, new initiatives, program priorities, previous commitments . . . other projected needs, and anticipated availability of funds."[7] In the end, then, the peer reviews may be heavily discounted depending on the priorities of the NCI and the Program Leadership Committee; the way they choose to focus funding can then affect the state of the art and what others perceive to be as important.

The Economics of the NCI

As the analysis of the NCI's budget in Chapter 2 demonstrated, neither the gross domestic product (GDP) nor the overall U.S. budget proved to be significant in determining the NCI's budget. Although this might reinforce the nonpartisan nature of cancer funding, it could just as well indicate political use of the NCI for pork barrel projects. One potential economic variable that could affect the operation of the NCI today is the Epstein allegation of conflicts of interest between the NCI and the pharmaceutical industry. In reviewing the biographies of the current NCI leadership (as of June 2016), those with available biographies had no overt ties to industry. In fact, most of the senior leadership of the NCI has spent a majority of their careers inside either the NCI or the NIH as professional researchers.

What about other parts of NCI? Although Epstein specifically indicts the President's Cancer Panel as beholden to industry, again as of 2016, none of the three members came from industry. The National Cancer Advisory Board, which serves in an advisory capacity to the NCI director, has only one representative from industry (out of a total of 17): Dr. William Sellers from Roche. The National Cancer Institute Board of Scientific Advisors, Board of Scientific Counselors (Basic Sciences), Board of Scientific Counselors (Clinical Sciences and Epidemiology), and the Frederick National Laboratory Advisory Committee have no members with industry affiliations. Only two advisory boards, the Clinical Trials and Translational Research Advisory Committee and the Council of Research Advocates, have members drawn from industry.

If industry does not have an impact on the NCI, at least not through the NCI's leadership and advisors, what impact can the NCI have on industry and the economy? The research that the NCI funds quite often leads to new ideas and drugs, which can be patented by their investigators; these patented drugs can lead to millions of dollars in profits for pharmaceutical companies, a piece of which the NCI does get in return. But these economic benefits do not just extend to large corporations; the NCI's Small Business Innovation Research (SBIR) and Small Business Technology Transfer (STTR) programs provide funding and support to small businesses with innovative research and technological innovations. And if those economic benefits weren't enough, the overall economy will ultimately benefit from having a workforce that is healthy and cancer free that can provide years of employment and new business ideas.

In looking at the political, social, scientific, and economic variables that might affect the National Cancer Institute, it would appear that the largest factors influencing their operations are scientific and social; what scientists do or don't know about cancer significantly influences what the NCI can and cannot do. A lack of public awareness of the NCI's activities may also influence their ability to get more funds or expand their activities; when the NCI has yet to be invoked in statements by Vice President Joe Biden about his moonshot effort to cure cancer, it shows just how little the public may recognize the NCI and its efforts.

Environmental Protection Agency

Created by Richard Nixon in 1971, the Environmental Protection Agency became the ultimate symbol of government response to the charges leveled by Rachel Carson in her book *Silent Spring*. Detailing the damage that pesticides were doing to the environment, Carson's book was a bestseller that helped lead to the broader environmental movement. The EPA was thus empowered by laws such as the Clean Air Act, the Clean Water Act, and the Toxic Substances Control Act to regulate the chemicals that were in our surrounding environment and that could come into contact with people. With the assent of the Carter administration, EPA regulators introduced hundreds of regulations involving chemicals in the late 1970s, many of which drew the ire of Republicans and business interests who saw the EPA as too active, thereby restricting the free flow of commerce and industry and stifling economic development. With the election of Ronald Reagan in 1980 and his installation as administrator Anne Gorsuch, the EPA's budget was severely cut and its activities significantly restrained. Since then, the EPA has remained a political football, either regulating too much or too little depending on your partisan bent.

So what does any of this have to do with cancer? Given that some people estimate that up to 50 percent of cancers are due to chemicals we encounter in our everyday lives, the way in which the EPA designs and implements regulations for potentially carcinogenic chemicals serves as a way in which the government enacts cancer policy and thereby helps to prevent occurrences of cancer. Aside from deciding what chemicals to regulate and how much to allow in the environment, the EPA has labored over standards through which they would be able to label a chemical as carcinogenic and/or toxic. These standards have become the focus of scientific and court battles alike as proponents and opponents challenge the decision-making of the EPA. While the EPA certainly isn't the only regulatory agency involved in protecting the American public from potentially toxic chemicals (OSHA is another), they are the most active in this area.

The Politics of the EPA

As numerous scholars have already detailed,[8] the EPA is a highly politicized agency. The most political aspect of this agency is the conflict between industry, which believes it is overly regulated, and those in favor of more stringently protecting public health. Making this even more complicated is the fact that the battle lines are not simply drawn during the regulation process itself—they can be found everywhere from the Congress and the White House to the courts. Although many would like it to be so, the regulatory process is not a closed one that focuses solely on the health costs of exposure to pesticides, waste, and air pollution, but rather is a process that invites democratic participation in which only a small few take part.

The debate between Republicans, who favor less regulation, and Democrats, who favor more, has been taken up previously in Chapters 1 and 2 so I will not replay the fight here. But there are two other political factors that can affect the EPA's regulatory actions: budgetary riders and the administrative law system under which it must act. To begin with, riders are policy statements that forbid an agency from spending money on a certain activity. These statements are attached by members of Congress to budgetary legislation, which is often "must pass" legislation. The number of riders that have been applied to not only the EPA but other agencies have only increased in recent years.[9] In prohibiting regulators from taking action in particular areas, legislators are controlling what regulators can and cannot do. To give an example of a recent policy rider that has been enacted, the EPA has been forbidden from enacting regulations on carbon production.

Riders are a controversial issue because budget bills are traditionally not used as vehicles for making policy. But in inserting a rider into it, the bill is promulgating official government policy. While there is nothing inherently wrong about the Congress, the people's elected officials, telling agencies what to do or not to do, the argument is over the way in which it is done. Because budget bills must be passed for fear of shutting down the government, riders are looked at as either a poison pill or a bitter pill to swallow. Further, critics of riders in environmental policy areas would argue that the proper place to evaluate the science of these regulations is in the agency itself, not by members of Congress who may be serving to protect entrenched interests in their district. However, that is what we ask our elected officials to do—represent the people who elected them in the first place.

The second political area, and perhaps the more consequential one, is the process of making regulations. Under the Administrative Procedures Act of 1946 and later legislation opening up the inner workings of government to the citizens, a number of public steps must be taken when creating and finalizing a regulation. First, an agency must give notice that it intends to make a rule or regulation and allow for public comment on the subject. After receiving these comments (if any are made) and reviewing the available research and data on the subject, the EPA or any regulatory agency draws up a preliminary regulation. This regulation is then published publically to give time for comment. Once the public comment period is over, they can either amend the regulation, depending on the received feedback, or finalize the rule. Even then, however, the process may not be over. If people or businesses still disagree with the regulation, they can challenge the agency in an administrative law court either over the data used to inform the regulation or the process through which the regulation was reached. Courts can order the regulation revised or rescinded, thereby opening up yet another avenue through which nonscientific opinions and information enter into the regulatory process.

Jasanoff, among others, credits this adversarial process with creating regulations that are designed to hold up to judicial scrutiny rather than scientific standards.[10] "The knowledge that their [the EPA's] decisions would be subjected to judicial scrutiny drove agencies to adopt formal analytical procedures, such as quantitative risk assessment, and to build massive technical records to satisfy judicial demands for 'reasoned decision making' and a 'hard look' at the evidence."[11] Because the EPA and other regulators know that their decisions are likely to be challenged by their opponents, they create elaborate systems, standards, and safeguards to protect themselves when the issue inevitably comes to the attention of a judge. It is for this exact reason that throughout the 1970s and into the 1980s, the EPA focused heavily on promulgating standards by which they would call a chemical carcinogenic or not. These standards became a battleground of their own, expanding from nine basic principles in 1976 to far more elaborate standards by the 1980s.[12] However, other agencies, including OSHA, the National Cancer Advisory Board, and Carter's Interagency Regulatory Liaison Group, also developed their own cancer guidelines thereby complicating conclusions about what would be considered dangerous.

The Social Side of the EPA

Much like the pesticide controversy stoked by Carson's *Silent Spring* that stimulated public outrage over the chemicals in their environment, regulation and the frequency of it can be seen as driven by public demand. Unfortunately, public concern with environmental regulations does not appear to be all that high, only rising when some sort of environmental catastrophe occurs, particularly in their own backyards. Instances of locally high cancer rates have often led local communities to demand answers and solutions, a pattern exemplified in the movie *Erin Brockovich*.

However, social concerns about the environment today are not oriented toward pesticides and other potentially carcinogenic chemicals that we face on a daily basis. Instead, public attention is devoted toward carbon pollution, renewable energy, fracking, and climate change. While these are certainly important issues, it simply means that the public clamoring and demand for chemical regulation is little to nonexistent. As we've seen time and again in American society, it often takes significant focusing events to bring the community together to demand changes.

The Science of the EPA

One of the elements that keeps dangerous pollutants and chemicals off of the worry list of most Americans is the scientific disagreement over the causes of cancer and whether they are in fact environmentally caused or not. This once again harkens back to the scientific dispute between the cancer establishment writ large and critics of their activities, like Samuel Epstein, who argue for a greater focus on prevention through the elimination of dangerous chemicals in the environment. If this continues to be a debate within the cancer establishment itself, how can anyone ever expect the public to jump on the issue and demand change? The scientific disputes can feed into a lack of social awareness and keep social demand for regulations low.

Similarly, most of the other scientific disagreements we've touched on previously also make an appearance in the fight over regulations. First of all, what kind of data is needed to demonstrate that a chemical causes cancer? Are experiments with animals sufficient or do you need to have evidence that cancer has occurred in humans who have been exposed to the chemical? If you use animals, can the cancer occur in only one type of animal, perhaps mice, or do you need evidence from multiple types of animals? And what type of exposure are you using on them at what level? These were the types of controversies that EPA regulators were attempting to sort out in establishing cancer guidelines as discussed earlier. However, industry can still criticize the methodology and the data used to determine dangerousness, often leading to protracted court battles that sap the EPA of their limited resources.

Early regulations established by the EPA fell victim to just these sorts of critiques. As a result, the EPA took two paths to shoring up their regulatory analyses: the first was the establishment of the cancer guidelines and a second was the creation of peer review and scientific advisory boards that the EPA could turn to verify and review their scientific data.[13] Since peer review, whether correct or incorrect, is viewed in the scientific community as the sine non qua of scientific standards, the EPA, if they could bring in and use peer review to their advantage, stood to gain scientific credibility in their promulgating of science-based regulations. Jasanoff details the establishment of their Science Advisory Board (SAB) in the 1970s with the job of "[r]eviewing and advising on the adequacy and scientific basis of any proposed criteria document, standard, limitation, or regulation under the Clean Air Act, the Federal Water Pollution Control Act, the Resource Conservation and Recovery Act of 1976, the Noise Control Act, the Toxic Substance Control Act, the Safe Drinking Water Act, the Comprehensive Environmental Response, Compensation, and Liability Act, or any other authority of the Administrator."[14] Made up of academics, public health officials, and members of industry, the SAB is a body that allows the EPA to claim scientific legitimacy in the wake of political criticisms. This does not mean that the EPA administrator is bound to take their advice into consideration. Jasanoff argues that the impact of SAB on EPA policy is difficult to measure but that its "prestige within the agency has grown over time."[15]

The Economics of the EPA

Perhaps one of the most important actors in the regulatory process is business and industry itself. Although the public comment period is supposedly to give the public an opportunity to express their opinion on the subject and therefore play a part in the democratic operation of this country, in studies of the regulatory process, Schotland and Bero and Bero et al. found that businesses and interest groups dominated in providing feedback and input into regulatory decisions.[16] In particular, industry-backed groups were primarily critical of the proposed regulations rather than supportive. They argue that this demonstrates not just that some agencies have been "captured" by those who they are in charge of regulating, but that even when regulations are finalized, business has an undue influence on their content and structure. Of course, it's easy to understand just why industry would be interested in regulations; banning a particular pesticide or requiring a particular level of technology to reduce wastes and pollution will have an economic effect either by decreasing profits or requiring greater investment in infrastructure. These economic effects are the primary argument used by Republicans against regulations and supposed overregulation.

The influence of industry can be seen in two other areas in the regulatory process: the writing and passage of budget riders and the legal adjudication process of the regulations. As alluded to before, members of Congress will often insert riders into budget bills to satisfy the desires of business interests in their states or districts. The members will often find themselves lobbied not just by the companies themselves but the lobbyists and special interest groups that represent them. According to the Center for Responsive Politics, in just the first half of 2016 alone, Pharmaceutical Research and Manufacturers of America had spent $5.9 million, Dow Chemical had spent $4.8 million, and both Exxon Mobil and Pfizer had spent $3.2 million each, all on lobbying efforts. This influx of money all but assures these companies will have a voice in the legislative process, whether in actual legislation or in budgetary matters, including the policy riders.

During the regulatory process itself, the companies and their lobbying firms not only have the opportunity to make their opinions heard during the public comment period, but they also possess massive resources to challenge regulatory decisions in the court. Because regulatory agencies like the EPA have a limited budget each year, they cannot engage in every lengthy court battle to defend every regulation they finalize. On the other hand, a company like Exxon Mobil does have the money and lawyers ready to battle the regulation in court. This gives a decided advantage to business and industry, particularly when judges have been less willing to give regulatory agencies the benefit of the doubt in scientific matters.[17]

The EPA is a highly politicized and democratized agency that has a substantial impact on cancer policy, but an agency on which others can also have a substantial impact. Politicians can actively limit the types of regulations they can promulgate, industry and interest groups have plenty of opportunity to have their views heard, and scientists are more often used to bolster and legitimize decisions rather than write them. For an agency that would want to undertake effective regulations for the prevention of cancer, these make formidable obstacles to establishing such rules.

The Food and Drug Administration

The Food and Drug Administration plays a two-pronged role in the fight against cancer: one, in ensuring that food additives and other components that we come into contact with such as packaging and processing materials are not carcinogenic and two, in reviewing and approving the drugs that are so vital in the fight against cancer. The FDA, as described in Chapter 1, is an organization that has grown in powers and responsibilities over time, as different constituencies and scandals have brought attention to the need to ensure safety in the food that all Americans eat. Similarly, the legislation enabling the FDA to act is a "product of incremental legislation action and administration adaptation," beginning with the 1906 Food and Drugs Act and expanded on in the Federal Food, Drug, and Cosmetic Act of 1938.[18] Importantly for our purposes, a key legislative provision was added in 1958 called the Delaney Clause. Named after Representative James Delaney who chaired a committee on chemicals in food, the clause states:

> Provided, That no additive shall be deemed to be safe if it is found to induce cancer when ingested by man or animal, or if it is found, after tests which are appropriate for the evaluation of the safety of food additives, to induce cancer in man or animal.

In effect, the Delaney Clause charged the FDA to ensure that no chemicals that could potentially cause cancer were allowed in the U.S. food supply; however, there were important restrictions on what the FDA could and could not oversee. The Delaney Clause did not and does not apply to all chemicals in all foods. Instead, it applies to food additives, a far more restricted category of chemicals. Further, the clause does not apply to substances that had been previously approved or sanctioned by the FDA or U.S. Department of Agriculture (USDA).[19]

In addition to regulating food additives and animal drugs that could be potentially dangerous to the human population, the FDA regulates prescription and over-the-counter drugs that many Americans take every day. In short, the FDA approves drugs both for clinical testing and after pharmaceutical companies have completed three phases of testing: phase I ensures the safety of the drug, phase II tests for effectiveness, and phase III is a large-scale test of effectiveness and safety focusing on adverse side effects. Once these studies are complete, pharmaceutical companies submit a new drug application (NDA) along with their clinical data for review. Although this process seems simple and straightforward, the decision making is anything but. Daniel Carpenter, in his authoritative study of the FDA in *Reputation and Power*, examines pharmaceutical regulation in great detail and argues that a primary driver of FDA decisions and actions is the preservation of their power and reputation.[20] This combination of pure power politics and science leads to a very complicated agency with its tentacles entwined throughout cancer policy and treatment.

The Politics of the FDA

Some of the political elements of the FDA have already been discussed previously, including budgetary and regulatory politics, so we will not dwell for long on these subjects. Obviously, when the FDA and other regulatory agencies are appropriated less money, they necessarily have fewer resources for enforcement actions and drug review. This goes not only for creating and enforcing regulations on food additives and medical devices but for drug review as well, which is an intensely employee- and resource-driven prospect. Over the past decade, the amount of money that Congress has appropriated to the FDA has steadily risen from $1.848 billion in 2006 to $4.359 billion in 2014.[21] Additionally, beginning in the 1990s, Congress imposed user fees on pharmaceutical companies submitting drugs for review while agreeing not to cut the appropriated funds for the FDA to provide the agency with more resources to allay some of the criticisms of delay and lag they were facing. While this would lead to fears of agency capture (which will be discussed later), the amount of money the FDA has to operate under has clearly risen.

Another political area in which the FDA has found itself involved is the language of rights, in particular, the rights of patients, doctors, and drug companies. In taking up the mantle of "gatekeeper" between drug companies and the American public, the FDA has inserted itself in a complicated dance between these actors, which has often been invoked to criticize the actions or lack thereof of the agency. Although we previously discussed the case of Laetrile in the 1970s, there have been other areas in which this battle has been fought, including HIV/AIDS and cancer drugs in general. In all of these cases, the general libertarian principles of little to no government intervention have come into play; proponents of the right-to-try movement argue that no one should be involved in treatment decisions but doctors and patients, and even then, patients should have the final say. Unfortunately, this rhetoric is most often invoked when the issue quite literally is life or death. If there is nothing left to try, then patients might be willing to try anything. In the case of cancer, this has most often played out in discussions of approval for trials of oncology drugs and their eventual availability to patients. Ultimately in the case of Laetrile, the FDA was sued in federal court over patient access to the drug absent the FDA's imprimatur. In the Supreme Court ruling in the case *United States et al. v. Rutherford et al.* (1979), the Court reaffirmed the power of the FDA to prevent unsafe or ineffective drugs from reaching the public market.

In addition to these usual suspects, Carpenter adds another dimension of politics to the discussion of the FDA, that of organizational politics. The main argument that Carpenter seeks to make is that the FDA has a historical propensity and need to protect its organizational image and reputation, as it is this reputation that gives it its power over the drug industry and drug manufacturers. A prime example of this phenomenon is the thalidomide controversy of the 1960s and the FDA's nonapproval of thalidomide, which prevented an outbreak of the heartbreaking birth defects that occurred in Europe following thalidomide's approval there. In the wake of the publicity surrounding the effects of thalidomide on babies, the FDA's Frances Kelsey, a medical officer in the Bureau of Drugs, found front-page fame as the woman who prevented thalidomide from being approved in the United States. As detailed by Carpenter, for years after, Kelsey was heralded as a hero and the FDA consistently looked at favorably by the American public.[22] Citizens saw the FDA as a legitimate protector of American health and safety and because the trust of the public was on the side of the FDA, both politicians and industry had incentive to respond to FDA actions and rulings.

Thus, the FDA must balance its responsibility to public health and safety with its responsibility to approve drugs that might be helpful to patients across America; unfortunately, this line is rarely as obvious as we might like it to be. Where exactly is that line in examining a drug or an additive that may be beneficial to people but causes side effects? And how bad do those side effects have to be to prevent the FDA from approving the drugs? These questions have led the FDA to require reams and reams of data and evidence from clinical trials, which are meticulously examined for possible problems with the drugs to be approved. What is ultimately at sake, for the FDA at least, is its reputation and power; if it approves a drug that proves dangerous to the public, it loses credibility in the face of the public and the politicians who oversee its actions. As a result, the FDA has often been called conservative in its actions.[23]

The FDA's pursuit of organizational and reputational power has often led it into conflict with another bureaucratic agency involved in cancer politics: the National Cancer Institute. With the increase in cancer drugs, particularly chemotherapeutic agents, under study in the 1970s, the FDA increased its scrutiny of NCI-sponsored clinical trials because of fears that these highly toxic chemotherapy drugs were causing more harm in patients than good. Because the FDA must approve clinical trials before they commence, FDA concerns often led to trial suspensions, which the NCI decried. The NCI believed that the cost/benefit calculation for dying patients was fair since these cancer-stricken patients were likely to die anyway without treatment; the FDA, however, only saw the intense and debilitating effects of the first generation of chemotherapy. Even before the HIV/AIDS battles of the 1980s, cancer drugs presented the FDA with a dilemma: Should there be any exceptions to the FDA's strict decision calculus based on the fact that the patients involved would likely die in any case?[24] Heightening the pitch of the fight was the fact that the FDA wasn't battling just any organization but another government agency.

Eventually, the heads of both the FDA and the NCI would negotiate a set of compromises both for oncologic drugs and their clinical trials. This does not mean, however, that the conflict between the NCI and the FDA has laid dormant ever since; in fact, some cancer researchers continue to decry two different aspects of the FDA, their consideration of surrogate endpoints during clinical trials, and the length of time it takes them to approve oncologic drugs.[25] For most clinical trials, the FDA requires that patients be tracked until an endpoint, usually death. However, for many drugs, including cancer drugs, it would be infeasible to wait to make the drugs available to patients if drug companies had to wait until every patient in their clinical trials died; as such, statisticians and doctors have introduced the concept of surrogate endpoints, or other standards by which success can be measured. In the case of cancer, these endpoints are often tumor response rate or length of survival. However, some researchers have been skeptical of these endpoints, arguing that they do not correlate with the success or failure of cancer drugs.[26] This ties into the second criticism of the length of time it often takes the FDA to approve oncologic drugs. In his analysis of approval times, Carpenter finds that between 1962 and 1985, oncology drugs had an average review time of 44 months, second only in length to neurologic drugs; from 1986 to 2004, this dropped to an average below 24 months.[27] However, a 2016 study showed that cancer drugs have the lowest chance of being approved by the FDA, with only a 5.1 percent chance.[28]

As a result of these conflicts between the NCI and the FDA, some proponents of the NCI have called for the NCI to take over approval of oncology drugs from the FDA, thereby threatening the organizational reputation of the FDA.[29] Clearly, these internecine battles between two different government agencies have shaped drug approval and cancer treatment, lending yet another political dimension to how we look at and treat cancer in the United States. In fact, politics within the FDA have become so entrenched that in June 2016, a group of former FDA commissioners, both Republican and Democrat, called for taking the FDA out of the Department of Health and Human Services and making it an independent agency.[30]

The Social Side of the FDA

In connection with the right-to-try movement, the social aspects influencing the FDA revolve around public awareness, activism, and patient politics. In taking charge of their own health, organized patient groups have pressured the FDA to approve drugs and even change regulations over drug approval, particularly with breakthrough drugs. This phenomenon has been particularly apparent in the AIDS movement and their push to have early AIDS drugs like AZT made available to those afflicted even before formal FDA approval. However, pressure has also been leveraged by other patient groups over topics including Laetrile, breast cancer, and cancer in general.

One aspect of this social pressure invokes the language of ethics and morality, particularly in the cases of cancer and HIV/AIDS. If, in early clinical trials, the drug under study showed promise in treating disease, activists argued that there were two ethical considerations to be taken into account. Traditional trial methodology measures the effectiveness of the investigational drug against the effectiveness of a placebo. The key to the placebo and treatment drugs is that the patient traditionally does not know which they are on. If the drug is proving successful, how is it ethical to provide some trial subjects purposefully with a placebo?[31] But if there isn't a control group, how would researchers know if the drug truly worked or not? Extending the argument to the second ethical point: What are the ethics of withholding it from any sufferer who wants it? Keeping a potentially lifesaving or life-extending drug from patients could feasibly result in the needless deaths and suffering of those affected. As a result of these critiques, the FDA has reduced its regulations for both proving efficacy and providing drugs preapproval for compassionate use.[32]

Public pressure, then, is a means to threaten the FDA with public disapproval should they behave in ways counter to the will of these organized groups. Indeed, Carpenter shows that the FDA moves quicker on drug approvals for those drugs that are considered to be new molecular entities when there is greater public attention focused on them.[33] Nonetheless, the FDA must balance the need to advance the drugs with protecting its own reputation. Many of the battles of AIDS drugs in the 1980s were influenced by the lasting legacy of both thalidomide and Laetrile; used in the rhetoric of the FDA, those two instances of failing to approve demonstrated the

caution and care that the FDA took toward the health and safety of prescription drugs in the United States.[34] Despite these examples of FDA effectiveness, AIDS activists quickly discovered that both protests and the threat
of protests would induce the FDA to approve drugs and approve them
quicker than normal.[35]

Social pressure in the form of organized patient movements or public
interest groups can be effective, but it is often difficult to achieve. This difficulty lies in many areas, not the least of which are the costs of organizing
on behalf of groups and individuals, including the free rider problem.
These groups also find it difficult to generate the requisite public awareness
needed to affect the FDA, short of some sort of focusing event like the AIDS
crisis in the 1980s or Nixon's declaration of war on cancer in 1970. Nonetheless, when it does happen, these instances demonstrate that social pressures are effective in influencing the FDA.

The Science of the FDA

Because of the nature of the work the FDA is charged with, science
plays an integral role in its decisions, and its decisions on what types of science to accept as valid influence the state of scientific work. As such, the FDA
is an arbiter, determiner, and provider of information through its gatekeep-
ing function for both food additives and drugs. While the image of "mid-
dleman" tends to be negative, the FDA provides this function, determining
what drugs reach American physicians and patients. From the perspective of the FDA, this is a critical function because of what they see as ill-
informed patients *and* ill-informed doctors.[36]

One of the key means through which the FDA influences the scientific
community is through the type of clinical trials and evidence they require
of drug developers and producers. Beginning in the 1960s after the passage the Kefauver-Harris Amendments to the Food, Drug, and Cosmetic
Act, the FDA began to issue guidance as to the types of evidence they
would accept as proof of a drug's safety and efficacy. Borrowing from the
guidelines of the National Cancer Institute, the FDA created the very
structure and language of clinical trials as we know them today: phases I,
II, and III.[37] Each of these phases would demonstrate a different aspect of
safety and effectiveness while looking for adverse effects. The general FDA
requirement of two randomized and controlled studies was also introduced
at this time. The effect of these requirements was to increase the scientific
rigor and standards of drug testing.

At the same time, the FDA's moves increased the status of pharmacologists in the fields of medicine and drug research and development.[38] The
FDA wanted pharmacologists involved not only in developing a drug but

in assessing things such as the body's metabolism of the drug and the biological mechanisms that are involved with changing the human body. As a result, drug companies increased the number of pharmacologists on their staffs along with statisticians and people involved in assuaging the FDA in the regulatory and approval process. Again, because the FDA held the power to approve drugs that would have huge economic benefits for these companies, drug manufacturers had huge incentives to comply with the FDA's orders and guidance on these issues. This does not mean that these standards were always accepted. Many critics in both research and development and the pharmaceutical industry pushed back against what they saw as draconian and unnecessary moves by the FDA. Although some of these cases challenged the FDA in court, the federal judiciary would largely affirm the FDA's powers, and the FDA's gatekeeper power would induce cooperation.

In realizing that their regulatory requirements were changing the face of science, the FDA also moved in the 1960s to create a large number of ad hoc and advisory committees to connect the agency to the wider scientific community.[39] Today, there are 33 advisory committees and an additional 18 subcommittees of the Medical Devices Advisory Committee. While these committees provide advice and opinions on approving drugs and medical devices, much of the ground work in preparing decisions is done by medical officers in the Center for Drug Evaluation and Research. What these committees do provide in addition to FDA connections with doctors and scientists is scientific legitimacy in the case of difficult or controversial decisions. This scientific legitimacy is crucial in defending the scientific reputation of the FDA and the types of research and data that it requires.[40]

As much as the science of drug research and development influences the decisions of the FDA, the FDA is just as influential on the state of science itself. FDA requirements and guidance shape the actions and behaviors of pharmaceutical companies that have billions of dollars riding on the decisions of the FDA. Decisions about the development of one drug over another and what might be approved by the FDA is significant in shaping drug research and development.

The Economics of the FDA

The fact that access to the U.S. market, the largest and most profitable in the world, is regulated by the FDA gives it an incredible economic power. Its decisions on the fate of a drug can lead to billions in profits or billions in losses. Huge shifts in the stock market value of pharmaceutical companies coincide with major FDA decisions and the release of phase I,

II, and III results in clinical testing. The fact that the United States is the only major developed country in the world that does not regulate drug prices or negotiate them down means that drug companies can place high prices and expect high profits on their blockbuster drugs.

The pharmaceutical industry has slowly come to accept this state of regulation by the FDA as it has evolved slowly since the 1930s and often as a result of public outcry over dangerous drugs in the marketplace. The concerns of the industry have generally centered around the twin concerns of overregulation and supposed government interference in the doctor–patient relationship.[41] As part of their regulations on labeling and marketing, the FDA must approve not only the drug, but also the primary and secondary indications for which it will be used. Although the FDA cannot stop off-label prescribing (or prescribing a drug for something other than its primary indicated use), the FDA can influence physician behavior in what they stipulate the drug should be used for. As a result, intense negotiations can erupt between drug companies and the FDA over the packaging inserts and labeling requirements.

Again, companies can and do push back in various forms. Although some companies have chosen to confront the FDA in court proceedings, pharmaceutical lobbyists can utilize well-placed political pressure as well. The threat of congressional hearings, investigations, or even legislation can affect FDA decisions. For example, following criticisms of a "drug lag" between Europe and the United States wherein some drugs are often available more quickly in Europe than in the United States, congressional investigations and other political and interest group pressure induced the FDA to change its approval behavior. In many years, the FDA will have a group of late December approvals as they rush to approve drugs by the end of the year and thereby increase their annual numbers.

Further, with the introduction of user fees in the 1990s and somewhat lax after-market reviews, some actually criticize the FDA as being in the pocket of the pharmaceutical industry. The imposition of user fees was ostensibly enacted by Congress to provide additional resources for pharmaceutical regulation and review; however, three fears have accompanied them. One, when user fees are paid, drug applications are placed on a so-called "fast track" requiring expedited FDA review. However, some FDA proponents fear that shortchanging the review could mean overlooking some potentially important data or information that may ultimately affect consumers. Two, in paying user fees, pharmaceutical companies may be able to "capture" the FDA or influence them into being more pro-business than pro-consumer. And finally, some fear that Congress would cut the funds being appropriated to the FDA because of the incoming user fees.

Although the Congress ultimately agreed not to, the fact that there is some sort of resource tie between business and the FDA could ultimately complicate regulatory matters.

In addition to the pharmaceutical industry, there is another group that is just as interested in the actions of the FDA: doctors. Surprisingly, doctors, as represented through the American Medical Association (AMA), have not always been entirely supportive of the FDA. Prior to FDA regulation of drugs, the AMA and its publications served as a clearinghouse for providing drug information to doctors. When the FDA moved to enter into this arena, the AMA initially resisted the FDA's efforts because it would have a negative economic effect on the AMA.[42] Further, the AMA saw itself as the provider of information to doctors, believing that the FDA should not get involved in the doctor–patient relationship.[43] While the AMA's obsequiousness would not be a major roadblock to the FDA's actions, it does raise the specter of the AMA and other doctors' groups as economic powerhouses just as involved in health care and cancer policy as the pharmaceutical industry.

The FDA is a complicated agency charged with even more complicated decisions. The decisions the agency makes have the potential to affect the health and safety not only of all Americans, but many people across the world. As such, all variables—political, social, scientific, and economic—are in play in discussing the role that the FDA has in cancer policy and cancer-related decisions. Just like many of the other topics we have come across already, although we would like to view the FDA's decisions as simply based in science and evidence, far too often different dimensions are involved and have the capability to influence the eventual decisions that they make.

The Regulations

One way in which we can examine the actions of these agencies is to look at the regulations they have enacted in regard to cancer. Because of the provisions of the Administrative Procedures Act, all federal regulations must be published in the *Federal Register,* which has put up all of their records online back to 1995. A search for all finalized rules containing the word "cancer" turns up over 2,500 documents; not all of these records are relevant, though. In order to complete this analysis, I examined each of these rules and classified them by agency and whether they loosened restrictions, tightened restrictions, or did neither. As an example, regulations that increased (either temporarily or permanently) tolerances for pesticides were considered as loosening restrictions whereas setting new limits on pollution or other chemicals that might be carcinogenic were classified as tightened. This allows us to not only examine overall frequency of regulations in accordance with the findings of previous scholars, but also to test whether regulatory burdens are lifted or enforced based on different factors.[44]

Between 1995 and 2015, there were 1,746 finalized regulations that could be construed as being used to reduce human contact with carcinogenic chemicals or agents. The vast majority of these (1,575) were written by the Environmental Protection Agency, as demonstrated in Figure 3.2, followed by the FDA and the Occupational Health and Safety Administration. Consistent with Hedge and Johnson's[45] findings, shortly after the Republican takeover of Congress in 1994, the number of regulations increased dramatically. In this case, the EPA went from publishing 20 regulations in 1995 to 32 in 1996 and 111 in 1997. When George W. Bush entered office in 2001, the total number of cancer regulations went from 85 to 83 and remained at an average of 78 throughout his two terms in office. What is most striking, however, is that in 2008, the last year of Bush's presidency, only 59 cancer regulations were enacted, which rose dramatically to 101 in 2009, the first year of Barack Obama's two terms in office.

There does appear, then, to be a partisan connection to the frequency of regulations enacted, with a lower average number of regulations per year

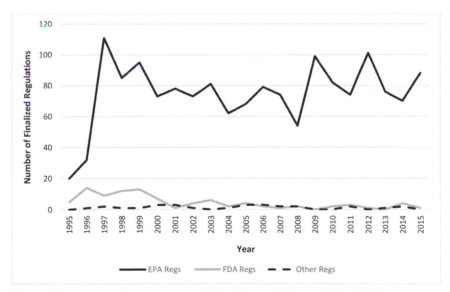

Figure 3.2 Cancer Regulations by EPA, FDA, and Other, 1995–2015 (regulations .gov)

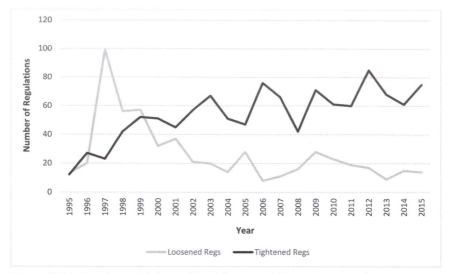

Figure 3.3   Number of Tightened Regulations and Loosened Regulations, 1995–2015 (regulations.gov)

during Bush's eight years versus an average of 86 during the Democratic administrations of Clinton and Obama. The trend does not seem to be apparent, though, in the strength of the regulations. Figure 3.3 shows the frequency of tightened versus loosened regulations between 1995 and 2015. From 1995 to 1998, the regulations that were enacted tended to be those that loosened restrictions; in particular, the bulk of these were EPA actions that temporarily raised pesticide limits in different crops due to different states of agricultural emergencies. For example, in 1997, the state of California petitioned the EPA to allow for the emergency use of the pesticide hexythiazox to control two-spotted spider mites on strawberry crops. Beginning in 1999, however, the frequency of these declarations decreased, and the regulations that were enacted tended to be those that restricted the use of or exposure to potentially cancer-causing chemicals.

Most of the new regulations that have been enacted by the EPA in particular are those that have been specifically requested by the agricultural and pesticide industries. A typical example is the case of the herbicide fluroxypyr. In 2006, fluroxypyr's manufacturer, Dow AgroSciences, petitioned the EPA to establish tolerance levels for the herbicide, which the EPA then did based on scientific studies provided to the EPA by Dow. Why would a pesticide or herbicide manufacturer actually *want* the EPA to enact restrictions? Sometimes, when action has been lacking by the EPA, states will enact their own limitations. When agricultural companies must deal with

50 different standards, they can incur high economic costs. It is more beneficial for them to have one federal standard enacted by the EPA, which they can request the EPA to do. The FDA is similarly subjected to petitions from industry asking them to certify food additives as safe and will often enact their own regulations as a reaction to the requests. If anything, this demonstrates the role of industry in influencing and making cancer regulations by requesting that the EPA act.

With respect to the FDA in particular, its low number of cancer regulations is surprising, particularly in light of the Delaney Clause and their specific responsibility to ensure the safety of the food supply. At the beginning of the series, the FDA was far more active in issuing regulations, averaging almost 10 per year from 1995–2000. After that, they averaged less than two per year, even after the Democratic president Barack Obama entered office. One possible explanation of this shift in behavior is the enactment of the Food Quality Protection Act of 1996; however, the timing of its passage does not seem to coincide with the change. Further, although the Delaney Clause used to be enforced by the FDA, most of its enforcement, particularly in the area of pesticides, was shifted to the EPA when it was created. What would be more important to the FDA, as we have discussed earlier, would be the approval or disapproval of oncologic drugs and the time period in which these occur. In an earlier study of drug approval times, Carpenter (2002) finds that drug approval times decrease when larger patient groups are involved and when there is greater media coverage of the drug. More recent analyses showing a slow-down in oncologic approval could also be indicative of FDA behavior, but this may also be a consequence of research and development choices made in previous years by pharmaceutical companies in either developing or not developing particular cancer drugs. In any case, the analysis here is too limited to be able to explain the shift altogether.

In sum, there are two major takeaways from this examination of cancer regulations. First, there is a distinct partisan flavoring in the frequency of regulations enacted, with far fewer being written during George W. Bush's Republican administration. Second, regulations are also influenced by industry; in fact, industry often prompts the EPA and the FDA to consider implementing regulations to begin with.

Conclusion

I considered an attempt at comparing the agencies discussed here, the NCI, the EPA, and the FDA, to determine which bureaucratic agency might have more influence over cancer policy in the United States. This, however, would be both difficult to do and highly unfair, as each of these agencies performs different functions in regard to cancer in the United States. The NCI contributes to how we think about and understand cancer as a disease and its treatments, whereas the EPA controls how much we may be exposed to potentially cancer-causing chemicals. The FDA regulates drug treatments and food safety, ensuring the chemicals that we are exposed to are as safe as could be expected given our exposure to them. Although these agencies often interact or even compete against each other for budgetary resources, all are instrumental in creating, enacting, and implementing cancer policy in the United States. And all are highly influenced by the political, social, scientific, and economic elements we have been discussing all along.

As difficult as it is to comprehend the level of politics involved in these three bureaucratic agencies, the power over these decisions does not stop here. Both the president and the Congress retain the ultimate leverage in influencing the behavior and activities not only of the NCI, the EPA, and the FDA, but of all government bureaucracies. It is to these two actors that we turn in the next chapter.

CHAPTER FOUR

Presidents Get Cancer, Too

Over time, great men (and women) of history tend to become abstracted figures to those of us living in the present. George Washington becomes the man who couldn't tell a lie, Abraham Lincoln the person who saved the Union. We forget that beneath all of the accomplishments and titles, beneath the fame and fortune, are people, men and women with feelings and desires just like the rest of us. They are imperfect, they are fallible. George Washington told many lies, and Lincoln often faltered in his drive to save the country. In forgetting about these vulnerable aspects of our greatest heroes, we lose a bit of their humanity, of the sense that we can be just as they were, warts and all. After all, presidents are people too.

And like all people, they have families and friends, people they care about and wish good things for. All too often, just like the rest of us, those loved ones suffer terrible misfortunes that presidents, people, must suffer through too. Cancer is just such a misfortune; it does not care whether you are looked at as a hero or villain, if you are famous or infamous, or if you are rich or poor. It is not discriminatory. It strikes as it will regardless of who or what you are. Presidents not only suffer the loss when someone they know has been afflicted by cancer, but they too can succumb to the chilling disease.

This chapter is about our modern American presidents: people, yes, but people in positions of authority and power as well. The *presidency* is something quite distinct from the *president*; the presidency connotes the office, machinery, and workings of the executive branch and the White House. The presidency includes the powers, the staff, and the constitutional abilities given to whatever individual happens to inhabit the Oval Office at a given point in history. The president is simply the person who, through the electoral process, is selected to serve in that office for a given period. The presidency lives on throughout the terms of the presidents and lives on when an individual president is gone and a new one comes to power. It is important to remember this distinction for if we take the person out of the presidency or the presidency away from the person, we lose the human connection that makes presidents just like us, albeit with more power.

Presidents get cancer and are just as likely to be affected by it as any other person in the country. Most of our modern presidents have had close family members who have been afflicted with various types of cancer, and one, Ronald Reagan, had cancerous lesions removed while he was in office. This very personal connection of arguably the most powerful person in the free world to a disease of this magnitude makes examining the issue all the more important. A president may never see war close up through the eyes of a loved one or a close friend, but they can see the suffering and consequences of cancer in themselves or their own family. We can imagine, then, that dealing with cancer up close can affect how presidents view cancer policy and therefore how they prioritize it. To examine these intimate and personal connections, this chapter proceeds as follows: first, we will discuss the position of the presidency with its attendant powers, responsibilities, and pressures as it relates to public policy in general and cancer more specifically. Then, we will examine the papers and statements of the post–World War II presidents and the rhetorical emphasis they have placed on cancer. Finally, we will break down the political, social, scientific, and economic pressures faced by presidents as they attempt to make and reshape cancer policy. As we will soon see, the personal impact of cancer is one that has left its dark and deep mark on many of our recent presidents.

The Pushes and Pulls of Being President

The president of the United States is a very different type of elected official, especially in the context of American politics. He or she is the only nationally elected politician, the only one who is ever voted on by the entirety of the country. In a way, this frees them from the constraint of localized constituent desires; they do not have to worry about the state of local roads or the closing of any given factory in Ohio or South Carolina. However, voters will still care about how presidents would respond to those types of issues. On the other hand, being president means that you must constantly worry about a whole host of other issues that other elected officials and their constituents might not necessarily worry about. For instance, if the country is to go to war or enter some sort of "conflict," a district without a large military base or military population might not care about it as much as a district with a military post in it. Even though a large number of voters might not care about the issue, war will almost always be at the top of the president's to-do list. The president faces a number of pushes and pulls toward and away from potential policy issues. In advantaging one over the other, the president appeals to different sections of the American electorate, but no one may ever be completely happy.

Another characteristic that makes the American presidency a different type of elected beast is the amount of responsibility and powers given to the person in the office. All too often, the American public views the president as close to all-powerful; this has certainly been disproved, however, in many cases. For example, although the president does have the ability to issue executive orders forcing the executive branch of government to do something or other, the ability to issue such orders is derived from and limited by legislation that has already been passed by the Congress and signed into law. The president cannot issue executive orders unless the power has already been granted to do so. The president may wish to go to war but the constitutional ability to declare war is given to the Congress. The president may wish to send troops into harm's way, but the Congress must ultimately pay for it and authorize it. These are but a few examples of how presidential power is significantly constrained by constitutional law and practice.

To be sure, the framers of the Constitution wanted it this way. Afraid of monarchical powers, they heavily circumscribed the powers of the president. And while a president's powers have grown since the establishment of the Constitution in 1789, it would still be a mistake to assume or make the argument that the president can do whatever he or she wants. Although the president may be able to do lots of little things, the big actions, the things that make the biggest difference, must be accomplished in concert with the Congress and the American people.

All of that being said, the president does have significant informal powers that he or she can use to influence the Congress and the voters and push them into agreeing with what he or she wants. In his classic tome on presidential power, Richard Neustadt argues that "[p]residential power is the power to persuade."[1] Because the president has so few formal powers, Neustadt says, they must use their rhetorical power and influence to make things happen; it is in this way that they exert influence and leadership over public policy in America. When Neustadt originally wrote *Presidential Power and the Modern Presidents*, he was writing in the context of the 1950s and 1960s, with presidents who could use their reputation to play "inside baseball" with politicos in Washington, D.C. Protecting one's image and reputation helped give the president an advantage with political rivals in D.C.; if other elected officials recognized the president's advantages, they would be more willing to negotiate or go along with what they wanted. With the advent of television news, the 24-hour news cycle, and particularly the Internet, presidents have the ability to "go public" today like never before. They have the ability to take their message to the voters and communicate directly with them. While research on the success of such a strategy is mixed (and not under the purview of this study), one of the president's most significant powers today is in public rhetoric and uses skills of persuasion.

Persuasion, power, and bargaining may indeed be tied up together, but another element that presidents must face in choosing how to use such tools is in choosing *when* to use those powers and on *what* issues. As the only nationally elected figure, presidents must respond to national and even regional or local crises. A president's failure to become involved or respond can mean peril and doom to one's presidency (for example, George W. Bush and his response to Hurricane Katrina in 2006). However, on any given day, there are innumerable problems and crises that presidents must respond to: mass shootings, overseas attacks, diseases like Ebola or Zika. And more often than not, when and how these crises appear cannot be controlled; events more often drive and control the president rather than the president driving and controlling the events. In the end, what presidents face is a seemingly unending list of ever-changing and ever-unfolding crises and only so much time in the day. Presidents must *choose* when and how to get involved in what situations, and those choices can signify the priorities of a president more than anything else.

Thus, presidents are faced with innumerable pushes and pulls; they are pushed to deal with events and crises that are beyond their control, they have limited amounts of formal power to do anything independently, they have other policy issues that they would like the American people and their elected officials to focus on, and they still only have 24 hours in a day. So what does any of this have to do with cancer policy? Even if a president *wants* to focus on cancer and make a policy statement, there are many other things in the day that cancer must trump in order for a president to do so. What tips the balance toward cancer? When does a president make that choice to spend the precious little time available to talk about cancer and persuade policy makers to make changes or take actions? In the modern era, that pressure has come in the form of political and social pressure, and unfortunately, personal experience.

One way to look at a president's rhetorical choices and therefore attempts at political persuasion is to look at when presidents have chosen to talk about cancer. Once again, if presidents choose to focus on it as a policy issue or policy problem, their statements can signal presidential determination to make a policy change. Fortunately, we have the *Public Papers of the President* through which we can search for such patterns. For this examination, I searched the *Papers* for mentions of the term "cancer" from 1945–2015. The initial search turned up 1,396 results. However, some caveats are in play. First, not every mention of "cancer" actually appears in the written statement; at some points, notes at the end of the statements say something about cancer and therefore the president never mentioned the term. Second, many mentions of "cancer" are in the context of the "cancer of communism" or "cancer of extremism," etc. These, then, are obviously not mentions of the disease cancer. Finally, not every statement that includes the word cancer is equal; if a president spends an entire speech or statement on cancer issues, that is obviously more significant than a president merely mentioning cancer in the context of a larger speech. As such, in examining these speeches, I classified each of the remaining 1,073 statements into one of the following categories: mentions, statements solely on cancer, and proclamations. The category of proclamations includes the annual proclamations by the president of National Cancer Control Month and, more recently, months and weeks dedicated to different types of cancer like cervical, breast, and colon.

The frequency of mentions of cancer far outnumbers the number of statements solely on cancer. Figure 4.1 shows the number of mentions of cancer in presidential speeches and papers from 1945–2015. The annual number varies anywhere from 0 to 79 in 2000 but averages to 12.28 mentions per

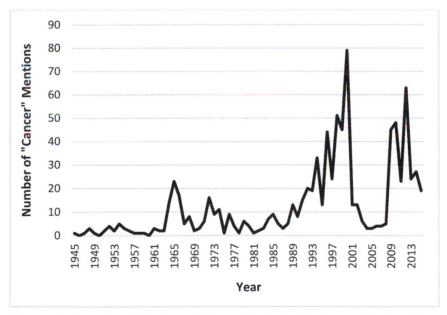

Figure 4.1   Number of Mentions of "Cancer" in the Public Papers of the President, 1945–2015

year. The number of mentions between 1945 and 1963 when Lyndon B. Johnson becomes president is fairly low. This is not surprising, particularly in light of the cultural taboo against talking about cancer or even mentioning the word. However, the influence of Mary Lasker, as detailed in Chapter 1, is exceedingly apparent during Johnson's administration; between 1964 and 1966, Johnson mentioned cancer 54 times and gave two speeches devoted to the issue, frequently invoking the story of his own mother, who died of cancer.

Johnson's focus on the issue of cancer is apparent when we compare the number of his mentions with those of Richard Nixon, who himself inaugurated the war on cancer in 1971. In Johnson's five years in office, he mentioned cancer a total of 67 times, whereas Nixon, in over six years in office, mentioned it 47 times. However, during 1971, the year in which he made his push for the war on cancer, Nixon gave eight speeches devoted to the topic, far more than any other president before or since. Even despite the war on cancer and Mary Lasker's efforts at pushing cancer to the top of the political agenda, the fact that these two men, brought up in the very time when cancer was looked at as a subject not to be discussed in public or good company, could even publicly mention cancer as many times as they did is important for breaking the social taboo and promoting the issue of cancer prevention and control.

While the number of mentions of cancer remains relatively high throughout the 1970s (an average of 6.6 mentions per year), an interesting pattern emerges. During Ronald Reagan's eight years in office, the average number of mentions drops to 4.3. Thus an interesting question emerges: Why would a man who himself experienced cancer and had a wife who also experienced cancer refrain from talking about the issue and promoting it? If the hypothesis of personal experience is to be believed, one would think that having such a firsthand experience with cancer would lead to a greater discussion or at least mention of it. What might be the cause of such a pattern?

There are two possible answers, neither of which can be substantiated within the scope of this project, but they are worth mentioning. One, perhaps Ronald Reagan, being older at his inauguration than previous presidents, was more inclined to adopt the cultural taboo of not speaking about cancer. Having grown up more fully in an age when that was not discussed may have led to a preference not to talk about it. However, previous presidents, including Truman, Eisenhower, and Johnson, who had all grown up and been socialized in a similar era, talked about cancer. A second, perhaps more plausible, answer is that being the oldest president elected to office at that time made Reagan and his administration more nervous about discussing potential health problems and dissuaded them from talking about Reagan's bout with cancer. Particularly given that Reagan had already survived an assassination attempt, the pressure to show that Reagan was physically able and up to the job trumped a willingness to discuss a malady that deeply affected both Mr. and Mrs. Reagan.

In any case, as is demonstrated in Figure 4.1, following the Reagan administration, presidents became far more likely to invoke cancer during their speeches. For George H.W. Bush and Bill Clinton, in particular, the mention of cancer became typical rhetorical flourishes on the campaign trail. For George H.W. Bush, the increasing number of mentions of cancer came in the context of the HIV/AIDS crisis. A typical statement at this time was that "we are spending a tremendous amount of money on AIDS, much more per capita on AIDS than we are on cancer."[2] We can attribute, then, the growing number of cancer mentions by George H.W. Bush not to an increased focus on the issue but to the growing criticism of the administration's response to the AIDS crisis. This is further supported by the fact that during his four years in office, Bush did not give any speeches solely devoted to the topic.

If Ronald Reagan was reluctant to speak about cancer, Bill Clinton was most certainly not. Having had personal experience with cancer (Clinton's mother, father, and uncle all suffered from it), Clinton did not shy away from using cancer in campaigning for health care reform in 1994, on the campaign trail in 1996, or to burnish his presidential legacy in 2000. In campaigning for health care reform in 1994, Clinton frequently invoked citizens' stories about experiences with cancer and the health care system to try to generate support for health care reform. A typical example has Clinton telling the story of someone with cancer who has met the lifetime limit on their insurance policy and must pay the remainder out of pocket or someone who had cancer and cannot get insurance later because it is considered a preexisting condition.

On the campaign trail in 1996, Clinton often used progress made on cancer research as a center point of his stump speech. In one such speech in Knoxville, Tennessee, he said:

> I just talked a little bit about health care, but technology is really making enormous strides there, and research is. During the time the Vice President and I have been in office, we've increased research on breast cancer at the National Institutes of Health by almost 80 percent. And just last year, an NIH scientist discovered two of the genes that cause breast cancer, giving hope for treating and preventing the second leading cause of cancer deaths among women.[3]

The genes Clinton mentioned in the speech were the BRCA1 and BRCA2 genes, and though he himself had not campaigned on such a platform, Clinton used these scientific advances to demonstrate the need for more health care research and even health care reform. He would also go on to claim the discovery of the BRCA genes as part of his presidential legacy in 2000, leading to the record high of 79 mentions of cancer in 2000 alone.

Surprisingly, just as cancer mentions quickly rose with George H.W. Bush and Bill Clinton, they just as quickly fell with George W. Bush in office. During his eight years in office, Bush averaged just 6.4 mentions of cancer per year, a surprisingly low total when compared to both Bill Clinton and Barack Obama who came into office after him. In thinking why this might be, previous hypotheses having to do with Reagan's pattern of mentions don't seem to be at play here; Bush did not grow up in an anticancer era, nor was he old enough that health problems might want to be downplayed. However, there is one major reason for cancer to recede on Bush's political agenda and that is the events of 9/11 and the subsequent war on terror. There is no doubt that the events in New York, Washington, D.C., and Pennsylvania that September day would become a prime focus for Bush and his administration; many of their domestic policy priorities would quickly be eclipsed by the war on terror. In fact, Bush's involvement in health issues and scientific research and development may have been higher given that less than a month before September 11, he gave a prime-time speech on stem cells and government funding for research using them (discussed further later). For a president to decide to give such a speech about medical research is significant and could have signaled the direction the Bush administration would take in their years in office. This would sadly change just a few weeks later.

The low number of mentions during Bush's time in office, however, stands in stark relief to the number of mentions by Barack Obama. In just seven years in office, he averaged 35.6 mentions of cancer annually. Although many of these came in the context of his health care reform, Obama frequently mentioned the deaths of his mother and grandmother, which were due to cancer, and their difficulties with the health care and insurance industries. This not only continues the presidential trend of invoking cancer in the cause of health care reform and crisis but illuminates the personal pressure and impact of having had a close relative suffer from cancer. While the year 2016 is not included in this analysis, the introduction of the "moonshot" to cure cancer with Vice President Joe Biden in the lead could just as plausibly continue the trend of high frequency of mentions.

In sum, these numbers certainly give us clues as to what influences the actions of presidents with regard to cancer. Personal experience with cancer appears to be a large driver, as does a push for health care reform. To explore these issues further, we now turn to examine the political, social, scientific, and economic elements that could influence presidential behavior.

The Politics

In examining the story of presidents and the politics of cancer, it is a story of response and rarely initiative. In the early decades of the 20th century, presidents rarely spoke about it; whether that was from the cultural aversion to talking about the dreaded disease or a lack of public pressure to do so is something that is hard to tease out. The earliest mention of cancer in the *Public Papers of the President* comes from William Howard Taft in 1910. The context is in a letter from the president to the Senate and the House forwarding a request for $50,000 to study cancer in fish. The justification for such a request, Taft writes, is as follows:

> The very great importance of pursuing the investigation into the cause of cancer can not [sic] be brought home to the Congress or to the public more acutely than by inviting attention to the memorandum of Doctor Gaylord herewith. Progress in the prevention and treatment of human diseases has been marvelously aided by an investigation into the same disease in those of the lower animals which are subject to it, and we have every reason to believe that a close investigation into the subject of cancer in fishes, which are frequently swept away by an epidemic of it, may give us light upon this dreadful human scourge.[4]

While it is not for the study of human cancers that Taft requests the money, he ultimately justifies it by arguing that the findings of such studies could provide enlightenment as to the causes of human cancers.

Following Taft's letter, the next mention of cancer comes in 1929 as President Herbert Hoover honored Marie Curie and mentioned how her discoveries had helped "[i]n the treatment of disease, especially of cancer."[5] Hoover again mentions cancer in the context of honoring Dr. James Ewing who "has done much to forward the attack upon the problem of cancer in particular and of disease in general."[6] Yet, none of these statements makes any mention of cancer in the political context, instead recognizing the works of individuals in relation to cancer.

The first political mentions of cancer begin in 1938 with President Franklin D. Roosevelt who associates the fight against polio (or "infantile paralysis") with the fight against cancer. In his radio address for the Fifth Birthday Ball for Crippled Children, Roosevelt states, "Today, the major fight of medicine and science is being directed against two other scourges, the toll of which is unthinkably great—cancer and infantile paralysis. In both fields the fight is again being conducted with national unity—and we believe with growing success."[7] Two facts stand out about this statement. One, it comes over a year after the establishment of the National Cancer Institute, the legislation for which Roosevelt signed into law. As we've discussed previously, the impetus for such an establishment was growing public and congressional pressure to do something about the rising rates of cancer in the country. Thus, Roosevelt's statement is not so much a presidential push for more attention to cancer as it is a reactionary statement recognizing that public awareness was already present. The second interesting characteristic about the statement is that it ties cancer in with another topic, in this case polio. Cancer as an issue does not stand on its own for Roosevelt, nor for his successors, Truman and Eisenhower.

Beginning in 1945 with President Harry Truman, cancer becomes tied to a different political issue: health care. In connection with his call for an economic bill of rights, Truman argues that "the health of this Nation is a national concern; that financial barriers in the way of attaining health shall be removed; that the health of all its citizens deserves the help of all the nation."[8] He then identifies five basic problems which he believes must be dealt with in order to fulfill his objectives; one of these is medical research and education under which he includes research on cancer. In the first public political argument about cancer made by a president, Truman states:

> Cancer is among the leading causes of death. It is responsible for over 160,000 recorded deaths a year, and should receive special attention. Though we already have the National Cancer Institute of the Public Health Service, we need still more coordinated research on the cause, prevention and cure of this disease. We need more financial support for research and to establish special clinics and hospitals for diagnosis and treatment of the disease especially in its early stages. We need to train more physicians for the highly specialized services so essential for effective control of cancer.[9]

Although it might appear that Truman is identifying cancer for special treatment, this paragraph is but one small part of the larger context of health care reform. Cancer continues to be tied to health care reform throughout the remainder of Truman's administration and even into the Republican administration of President Dwight D. Eisenhower. For President Eisenhower, cancer is also tied into health care reform, and he continued to call for greater funds for cancer research and treatment.

We must keep in mind that at the very time Truman and Eisenhower were making more calls for increased funding, the American Cancer Society and Mary Lasker were hard at work publicizing the issue of cancer. Given the discovery of the Salk vaccine and the eradication of polio, Lasker wanted cancer to slip in and fill the void left by a cured disease. Thus, it is certainly understandable that presidents would react to such public awareness and at a minimum continue the calls for more research and understanding into the disease.

The ultimate success of the ACS and Lasker would not come until the administration of Lyndon B. Johnson, with whom she had a close, personal relationship. We can clearly see Lasker's influence in the statements of Johnson, who often praises Lasker and recognizes the work of the ACS. Although the number of cancer mentions decreases toward the end of his term, we can infer that the pressure of the war in Vietnam was taking up more and more of his time; given those political pressures, it's understandable if, even if he wanted to, he was unable to push for anything further with respect to cancer. That task would be left to President Richard Nixon with his declaration of the war on cancer. Since we have addressed Nixon's policy agenda with respect to cancer elsewhere, suffice it to say here that Nixon, like the presidents before him, was responding to political and interest group pressure to do something about the growing number of cancer victims. Although historical counterfactuals are always difficult and near impossible to prove, an argument could be made that without Lasker and the ACS pushing for Nixon to "end cancer," Nixon might never have taken the ultimate step in calling for a stepped-up effort against the disease.

As we move into the 1980s, cancer unfortunately gets caught up in the regulatory politics and attitudes of the Reagan administration. As detailed previously, Republican presidents tend to be antiregulation. It's not that they're pro-cancer; in fact, they probably don't even connect the two issues together. Reagan's antiregulatory posture combined with his reluctance to talk about cancer despite his own battle with it (discussed in more detail later) put cancer policy on the backburner throughout the 1980s, with efforts at preventing cancer through regulations suffering along the way.

Despite this, the 1980s were a crucial period in other respects. New health issues arose, including HIV/AIDS, which would entangle with cancer issues. Second, modern political campaigning and the media were rapidly changing; presidents were increasingly expected to be more available, and 24-hour news networks had the pressure of filling the long hours of the day. These characteristics combined for increased mentions of cancer in a very political context. Barnstorming presidents, campaigning almost nonstop throughout the fall of election years, must make many, many speeches; instead of writing a new one for each campaign stop, a generic stump speech is used, perhaps altered somewhat by the location and news of the day. Beginning with George H.W. Bush, cancer makes its way into these stump speeches, but why? Claiming progress on cancer research or calling for increased efforts to cure cancer is good politics; who's going to be against such policies? As an example, in one such public town hall event leading up to the 1992 election, Bush is asked about spending on AIDS compared with other priorities. While recognizing that spending on AIDS had doubled, Bush argued against further increases, asking about cancer and other health issues that must be balanced along with that.[10] Thus, the president is balancing two very difficult political issues, HIV/AIDS and cancer.

President Bill Clinton's statements about and mentions of cancer bring together all of these political patterns. Not only did Clinton connect cancer with health care reform, making a stunning number of mentions of it in 1994 as he campaigned in the midterms and for his health care effort, he also used cancer as a political tool on his way to reelection in 1996. In the spring of 1996, Clinton called for an "Anticancer Initiative" with four major proposals: accelerate cancer drug approval, expand access to drugs already approved in other countries, better representation for cancer patients in FDA advisory meetings, and fewer applications for additional uses of approved cancer drugs.[11] This proposal is interesting in that it doesn't necessarily call for more resources but contains many actions that the president could undertake on his own either through regulatory reform or other executive action. Later in 1996, Clinton expanded on these proposals in announcing greater support for genetic research, a new national website for information on breast cancer, and recognizing that legislation that was passed would not allow insurance companies to deny coverage to cancer survivors.[12] Once again, easy moves to campaign on that hardly anyone could object to.

Despite the fact that Clinton's proposals could be easily followed through on and did not constitute any new major steps forward in the fight against cancer, Clinton still used such changes to help burnish his presidential legacy as his administration ended. Throughout 2000, Clinton touted revolutionary breakthroughs such as the discovery of the BRCA1 and BRCA2 genes and the passage of the Patients' Bill of Rights, which affected insurance coverage for many people, including cancer patients. The large number of mentions is evidence not just of the volume of campaigning that modern presidents have come to be expected to perform, but the extent to which Clinton claimed many of these cancer advances to be his own.

As noted earlier, George W. Bush did not make much of an issue of cancer during his term in office, and a possible reason for this will be discussed later. The same cannot be said of President Barack Obama, who, like Clinton, has also used cancer in pushing for health care reform and shaping a postpresidential legacy. Like Clinton's cancer-related arguments in favor of health care reform, Obama argued, among other things, that health care reform would lead to better treatment and outcomes for cancer patients. Frequently invoking the experience of his mother who died from uterine cancer, Obama cited the incredible worries and paperwork burdens that she had to experience. Obama would also use stories of cancer patients that he received to support reform. One such story comes from a speech on health care reform in 2009:

> And I—every day I get letters from people. I just got a letter two days ago from a woman who had been changing jobs, had just gone to sign up for her new Blue Cross Blue Shield policy, but in January, before she had taken her new job, she had felt a lump and had been referred to do a mammogram and found out, unfortunately, she had breast cancer. Well, the new insurance policy just said, this is a preexisting condition; won't cover it. She now owes $250,000.[13]

Clearly, cancer is personal for Obama, but it also hit close to home for his vice president, Joe Biden. In 2015, Biden's son, Beau, died of brain cancer at the age of 46. Given the timing and incredible loss, Beau's death kept Biden from running for the Democratic presidential nomination in 2016. But it also influenced both Biden and Obama to carry out a larger effort against cancer. In his 2016 State of the Union, Obama called for a new "moonshot" effort to cure cancer, with Biden as its head. While it was only a small part of the speech and short on details, Biden took the lead right away, promoting new policies aimed at speeding a cure. That night, Biden posted an essay online describing two major priorities of the policy push: increase resources and "break down silos" to increase the flow of information across all stakeholders.[14]

Unlike many initiatives, the White House did not just give lip service to the effort; throughout 2016, Biden has continued pushing the initiative with the White House, sponsoring a "pep rally" of "more than 270 events aimed at boosting support for the effort to speed up cancer research."[15] The event brought together government agencies like the NCI and the FDA with private companies like IBM to ease communication and research ability across the cancer community.

Although Obama's and Biden's efforts continue, it is worth noting the interesting rhetoric of the plan. Instead of using the term "war on cancer," which has been in use since Nixon, Obama and Biden have chosen the term "moonshot." Why the different language, and what might be the significance of such a shift? Unfortunately, when the term "war" is used in any sense, whether it's a war on cancer, war on drugs, or war on terrorism, the inevitable question is: Are we winning or losing? Indeed, the war on cancer has been subject to intense criticism with many people arguing that we have lost. In choosing the term moonshot, Obama and Biden can avoid such unfortunate usage while invoking a glory period of American research and development: the Apollo program and the eventual moon landing in 1969. The hope, then, is like the Apollo program at NASA before it, a moonshot effort to end cancer can focus an intense amount of energy and resources over a short period of time to make progress in the fight against the disease. In this case, then, even the choice of political rhetoric is calculated to avoid negative connotations and promote positive ones.

In looking back at presidential politics and cancer, cancer has historically been tied to other issues, most prominently health care reform. Presidents have tended to be reactionary to public and political pressure but also influenced by personal battle scars. Finally, the politics of cancer are such that it rarely will find an enemy; in this sense, cancer is a "safe" issue to both campaign on and claim as a presidential success.

Social Pressures

In discussing social pressures previously, we've generally talked about public opinion and awareness of cancer issues and the societal pressure to do something about the epidemic. In the case of the presidents, however, social pressure is really personal pressure; personal experience with cancer appears to intensify, or rather prime, presidents' political behavior toward it. To be sure, there is a major exception to this argument, that of Reagan, whose own occurrence of cancer did not seem to lead to any radical change in the president's behavior toward cancer.

In looking back at the personal experiences of the men who have held office, however, it is intriguing to identify their individual experiences and then look at their political action. Presidents Truman, Eisenhower, and Kennedy had no previous personal experiences with cancer (by which I mean either suffering from it themselves or having a close relation with cancer). John F. Kennedy did have other medical experiences from which to draw, primarily the case of his sister, Rosemary, who received a lobotomy at the age of 23. During his presidency, Kennedy would champion issues surrounding mental health, signing legislation creating community mental health centers and largely doing away with government support for sanitariums. In the postwar period, Lyndon Johnson would be the first president with firsthand experience in watching a family member suffer from cancer—in this case, his mother. Although he gave no details, in a speech launching the 1966 Cancer Crusade, Johnson said, "The loneliest moment I ever had in my life was when I learned that my mother was gone from me, because of this terrible disease."[16] His personal experience combined with the lobbying of Mary Lasker and the ACS would both contribute to Johnson's dedication to the issue of cancer and his numerous statements on it. Richard Nixon had no previous personal experience with cancer, but his declaration of a war against it can be seen as a culmination of the work of Lasker and the ACS and the groundwork laid by Johnson in the years prior.

While cancer receded as an issue in the mid to late 1970s, both presidents of that time period, Gerald Ford and Jimmy Carter, had situations where cancer hit close to home. For Ford, it was his mother and his wife, Betty, who underwent a radical mastectomy during Ford's time in the White House. Choosing to be open with her battle with breast cancer following the cover-ups of the Nixon administration, Mrs. Ford's openness about her cancer would lead to an increase in self-screening and therefore to an increase in women discovering they had breast cancer.[17] Despite the increase in incidences, Ford's public battle with breast cancer most likely led to millions of women receiving treatment earlier in the course of their disease. Clearly, Mrs. Ford and her health battles not only with cancer but also addiction led to an increase in public awareness and public discussion about topics that were previously considered to be taboo; however, her openness also led to better education and knowledge on the subject, which changed the way many Americans thought about and dealt with such issues.

This brings us to the case of Ronald Reagan. At the age of 69 when he was sworn into office, Reagan was the oldest person to become president at that time. When he was shot just months into his presidency, the thought of an early death for the oldest president became all too real. Likewise, when Reagan announced he was having surgery to remove a polyp in his colon in 1985, the question about death and ability reared its head once again. In an interview with Hugh Sidey of *Time* following his cancer treatment, Sidey specifically asked Reagan about the possibility of his resignation if the cancer recurred and Reagan would have to undergo any further treatment. Reagan replied,

> I can't foresee anything of that kind, and that is not just me talking, now. That's on the basis of all that I've been told by the doctors who were all involved in this. I can't see anything of that kind coming. But, as I said once when they were talking about my age before I was elected the first

time, if I found myself ever physically incapacitated where I, in my own mind, knew I could not fulfill the requirements, I'd be the first one to say so and step down.[18]

Reagan's discussion of his age and potential disabilities in office is interesting for the fact that Sidey did not invoke his age in the question, merely his ability to continue in office should he need further treatment. This demonstrates that Reagan was well aware of public and political concern about his age and health and his desire to downplay any such arguments, even in his second term.

While Reagan's attitude toward his cancer seems cavalier in a sense (in the same interview, he continually downplayed the threat of the disease in reiterating that he *had* cancer), his own previous personal experience with cancer could be indicative. In the Sidey interview, Reagan stated, "I've got too many friends—even my brother who—good Lord, he had very severe cancer of the larynx. He was a very heavy smoker, which I have never been. But that was golly, I guess in the neighborhood of 20 years ago, and he's doing just fine."[19] Thus, what Reagan had personally known of cancer was that people could easily survive even severe cases and that many people he knew who smoked were just as fine. All of this goes into his downplaying of the threat of his health and likely the threat of cancer in general, even after his wife, Nancy, underwent surgery for breast cancer in the next year.

This is not to say that his health scare had no impact whatsoever. Brown and Potosky show that Reagan's experience with cancer did lead to a change in public awareness.[20] Among other findings, they report an increase in calls to the NCI's Cancer Information Service as well as an increase in the number of people seeking tests for early detection of colorectal cancer. The caveat to these findings, however, is that these increases were only temporary and resided quickly once the episode was over.

Unfortunately, all of the presidents who have so far come after Reagan have had personal brushes with cancer. George H.W. Bush's father and George W. Bush's grandfather, Prescott Bush, died from lung cancer, Bill Clinton's parents and uncle had it, and Barack Obama's mother and grandmother died from cancer. For both Bill Clinton and Barack Obama in particular, their experiences watching someone close suffer from cancer would bring a personal touch to their respective campaigns for health care reform as they often invoked their own experiences to justify reform. Although George H.W. Bush certainly mentioned cancer a number of times, he did not use his father's death in justifying any changes in cancer policy. Similarly, George W. Bush did not summon the memories of his grandfather's death in his discussions of cancer, which were considerably fewer in number than either Clinton or Obama. In the case of George W. Bush, it is most likely the case that there was simply no room on the agenda to deal with cancer when concerns were higher about terrorism and homeland security. However, there is some evidence, discussed later, that had 9/11 not happened, Bush might have taken on health issues in a very different manner.

It is easy to see, then, how earlier life experiences can prime presidents to view issues in a particular light. This is the case not just for cancer, but for many other policy areas that presidents are expected to deal with. It's also true for the rest of us in our everyday lives. In this sense, these personal experiences bring home to us the very real humanity that confronts even the most powerful people on earth and their helplessness in facing a disease that simply does not care about status.

Scientific Pressures

Of the many items that reside on a president's agenda, science or scientific issues rarely make it to the top. The economy, foreign affairs, and whatever happens to be making the news that day crowd out the "less important" issues, which are left for other people to deal with. For something like cancer to make it on to the president's agenda signifies that a great deal of public and political attention is being focused on it. As we have seen so far, public awareness and political pressure interacting with a president's own personal experiences appear to influence when presidents talk about cancer and how they do so. However, one major limiting factor is the state of scientific knowledge.

Presidents cannot force scientists to come up with new ideas, groundbreaking findings, or advance the study of anything, let alone cancer. What scientists and doctors are able to do in the moment can also condition what policy statements presidents call for at a given time. It would not make any sense for a president to call for something that the scientific community cannot deliver on; presidents want to make policy promises that are deliverable and achievable so that he (or she) can claim the credit for making those innovations. If a president calls for something that is impossible, it can only hurt them down the road for being unable to fulfill the promise. Nobody but Nixon could have called for a war on cancer because the science had yet to advance enough to allow him to do so.

In this sense, the state of the art influences presidential actions, and 1971 is a perfect period to examine this scientific zeitgeist. As discussed in Chapter 1, the post–World War II period was an era of science and the science of the possible. The manned landing on the moon in 1969 is the prime example of this; the call heard around the country was "If we can land a man on the moon, we can do x." In fact, Nixon himself was very excited by the possibilities coming out of such an achievement. Not only did he look at the astronauts as heroes and symbols of scientific and American prestige, he was also a fan of the agency who had put them there, NASA.[21] While budgetary circumstances precluded Nixon from calling for a more expansive post-Apollo program for NASA, Nixon enthused about the prospects that an agency like NASA could do for the rest of America. At one point in the early 1970s, Nixon proposed to his staff that NASA be turned into an agency of problem solvers which would be given incredible technical challenges and be expected to come up with solutions to them.[22] This demonstrates not only Nixon's support for scientific achievement but his belief that it could be done.

It is not hard to imagine that Nixon's trust in scientific advancement could have influenced his call for a war on cancer. The postwar enthusiasm for science combined with the political and social pressure made it easy for Nixon to call for a war on cancer. In fact, a team of scientists from NASA was sent to the NCI in order to assist them in Nixon's new policy idea. If Nixon did not think such a thing was possible, it's not likely that he would have gone out on a limb to call for it. However, as we know now, the science surrounding cancer certainly did not develop as quickly as Nixon thought it would in 1971, and within a decade people were questioning whether the war on cancer could ever be truly won.

The fact that the science of cancer did not advance quickly would leave future presidents with a bad taste in their mouth for relying on the process of scientific advancement. This is evident in the anticancer proposals that Bill Clinton put forward in 1996; none had to do with encouraging scientists and doctors or calling for a cure. Instead, they were focused on process, regulations, and information. The rhetoric of war and the inevitable win/loss discussion that would follow would make for a difficult precedent to follow, as no president would want to be the one who "lost" the war on cancer, regardless of whether the president could actually influence the science or not.

Although not pertaining to cancer directly, another example of how the state of science has influenced presidential decisions was George W. Bush's decision on stem cells and their usage early in his administration. Throughout our body, different body parts are made up of different types of cells: skin cells, liver cells, blood cells, etc. Stem cells are cells that are capable of becoming any type of cell in the body and are important for many different research programs from Alzheimer's to cancer. What is controversial about stem cells is that they are derived from human embryos, and many conservatives argue that using such embryos for research is tantamount to abortion. In a televised primetime address, Bush made the announcement that federal funds would not be used to create new stem cell lines from embryos but could be used for research on already existing stem cell lines.

Reaction to Bush's decision was largely split down the middle, with many conservatives hailing the decisions and scientists decrying it. One prominent Republican who criticized the decision was Nancy Reagan, whose husband was by then suffering from Alzheimer's disease. Because of the research that could be done on curing or treating Alzheimer's, Mrs. Reagan was vocal in her opposition to the move. Despite this, what is interesting about this episode was that George W. Bush took his very valuable presidential time and energy to give a primetime speech on this issue. Why did this issue make it to the president's desk at that point in time, and why was it given such a high priority by the administration?

With the advent of cloning and more sophisticated means of genetic manipulation and research and the amount of government support that scientific research gets, it became an important question in 2001 to decide the limits on government support and funding for such endeavors. With a conservative Republican as president, the issue of whether stem cell research was killing fetuses became a political topic, and in a pre-9/11 era, these types of issues could easily come to the forefront. Bush's decision on stem cells is yet another example of a president reacting to scientific developments and making policy decisions based on the state of scientific advancement.

All of this leads to Obama and Biden's moonshot to cure cancer. While it is certainly motivated by personal loss and political prestige, it, too, is influenced by what science can and cannot achieve in the early decades of the 21st century. To that end, many of the activities the moonshot is undertaking are those to enhance scientific cooperation and communication not only across and between doctors and researchers, but with patients as well. Additionally, more emphasis is being placed on genetic components of cancer, something that can only be done with the technology of today. Once again, then, it is an example of how presidents can only use the science that they have in making policy proposals, not the science they wish they already had.

Economic Pressures

Because of their status as a nationally elected representative, presidents are somewhat immune from the day-to-day variances of local economies. Their concern is for the greater economy as a whole, and so their economic ties to the country are likely to be quite different from members of Congress, who we will discuss in the next chapter. One area in which we may be able to see economic and business group pressure play out is in the nature of the appointments presidents make to important positions. This, in fact, has been one criticism of Epstein and his colleagues, that interest groups like the American Cancer Society and other boards have too much influence from business. While we largely debunked that claim in the previous chapter, one other way we may be able to infer industry influence is through whom the president has appointed to his cancer panel.

The President's Cancer Panel (PCP) was established in 1971 in the National Cancer Act and consists of three members who oversee the national cancer program and report to the president on its activities. Its members serve staggered three-year terms with the option of reappointment. In examining the biographies of the men and women who have served on the PCP, six have connections to either industry or major interest groups (Table 4.1). Both Nixon and Reagan appointed members with strong ties to industry, in the case of Nixon, Benno C. Schmidt, and for Reagan, Armand Hammer. In later years, George H.W. Bush, Bill Clinton, and George W. Bush nominated members who had ties to the interest group community. However, out of the 25 people who have served or are currently serving on the PCP, the number of members with industry and interest group ties is fairly low. Further, there is no clear evidence of a difference between Republican and Democratic presidents except to say that the two members who were appointed out of industry were both appointed by Republicans.

Table 4.1   Appointments to the President's Cancer Panel with Ties to Industry or Interest Groups

Member	Nominated By	Industry Connection
Benno C. Schmidt (chair)	Nixon (1972)	Lawyer and venture capitalist; invested in fertilizers
Armand Hammer (chair)	Reagan (1982)	President and CEO of Occidental Petroleum Corp.
Nancy C. Brinker	H.W. (1991)	Chair of Komen Foundation
Harold P. Freeman	H.W. (1991), reappointed by Clinton	Past president of the American Cancer Society
Frances M. Visco	Clinton (1993)	President of National Breast Cancer Coalition
Lasalle D. Leffall	W. Bush (2002)	Past president of the American Cancer Society

One area of potential economic impact with respect to presidents and cancer is in the area of oncologic drugs and specifically, the government's ability to negotiate lower prices for them. "Proponents of government negotiation argue that HHS [Department of Health and Human Services]—because of its significant purchasing power—can more effectively negotiate drug prices than individual part D plans. Opponents argue that allowing the government to negotiate prices for Part D would inhibit innovation and limit beneficiary access to medications."[23] Prior to George W. Bush's introduction of a drug benefit to Medicare plans in the early 2000s, the biggest political football was simply the establishment of a drug benefit. Although he recognized rising prescription drug costs, Bill Clinton did not go so far as to call for the federal government to have the ability to negotiate with drug companies on drug costs. The same went for George W. Bush when Medicare Part D was initiated.

What is key to understanding this controversy is that the United States is one of only a handful of industrialized democracies who do not negotiate lower drug prices on behalf of their citizens. Given this, pharmaceutical companies know that they can make more money in the American market and therefore plan their research, development, and marketing around such an economic windfall. With pharmaceutical companies investing heavily in lobbying, topping out at over $272 million in 2009, politicians have been reluctant to call for, let alone support, negotiations with pharmaceutical companies.

One other primary reason that the Obama administration in particular has been reluctant to tangle in such an area is the politics surrounding health care reform. In 1993 when Bill Clinton asked his wife Hillary to work on a health care reform plan, Mrs. Clinton's efforts were largely conducted behind closed doors with little to no input from interest groups or industry. When her plan was released, it immediately attracted criticism not only from industry but from major interest groups like the American Medical Association. In fact, a consortium of interest groups collaborated on the famous "Harry and Louise" commercials, which helped to sink public opinion and support for reform. Learning from these mistakes, the Obama administration encouraged interest group and industry involvement in writing the 2009 reform package that would become the Affordable Care Act. In courting these actors, the administration was able to guarantee their buy-in and support; in fact, a group of interest groups got together again for a set of commercials bringing back the Harry and Louise characters, this time in support of health care reform.

Thus, the economic and political pressures to avoid policies such as drug negotiation are quite high. Regardless of whether individuals from these areas are appointed to key positions or not, larger policy goals—in this case a Medicare drug benefit or larger health care reform—were primary to attempts to lower drug prices through negotiation.

Conclusions

Whether we make them out to be good, bad, powerful, weak, or even a hero (or antihero), presidents at the end of the day are human. They suffer the stress of having to make life-or-death decisions on a daily basis. They make the most difficult decisions that many of us would never want to make. Cancer can just as easily affect these supposed superhumans as it can affect any one of us. And when it does, it can serve as a lasting influence for people in immense power to try and use their influence and persuasion for the better in terms of cancer policy.

This doesn't mean that cancer doesn't get tangled up in myriad other political issues; it most certainly does. As we've seen in this chapter, cancer is usually tied into other health policy issues, most prominently health care reform. It's often pursued in response to public pressure or lobbying like that of Mary Lasker. It's conditioned on what science can actually achieve at that moment in time and other competing priorities of the president. Or it might be avoided altogether when trying to avoid bringing health issues to the forefront of society's mind.

While presidents can try to achieve better cancer policy, it is important to remember Neustadt's admonition that presidential power is often limited to the power to persuade; the power to make other people want to do what you want them to do. What presidents can achieve alone is significantly limited and dependent on other actors in the political world. Others are involved to achieve the big policy goals, most prominently Congress. We next turn to examine the world of Capitol Hill and the very different types of pressures that members of Congress are likely to face.

All Cancer Is Local

If there is anything more hated than cancer, at least in recent years, it might just be the U.S. Congress. The institution has become synonymous with doing nothing and talking big. In some public opinion polls, trust in the Congress has fallen into single digits, with colonoscopies being rated as more preferable. But there is a conundrum here; for all of the griping, bellyaching, and lambasting of Congress, members are facing a reelection rate hovering around 90 percent. If Congress is so terrible, why are we not voting the bums out of office and replacing them with people we feel can get the job done? This is a well-known phenomenon in political science— voters believe that the Congress as a whole is terrible but absolutely love their own representatives.

While the reasons for this phenomenon are plenty, one major argument supporting it is that when representatives go back to their district or state, they can claim to have done something special for their constituents, whether it's securing funding for road repairs or changing tax policy that will save many of them money. Or what about money for a fire engine that will now have that member's name emblazoned on it? In past years, this was called "bringing home the bacon" or more simply pork barrel spending. In Congress, opportunities abound for members to secure for themselves and their voters the benefits of public policy. While the Congress as a whole may fail to pursue large policy outcomes or even legislating, members can often be successful in chasing the goodies for their friends and neighbors.

Why should it be any different with cancer? Despite its national prevalence as the second-biggest killer (second only to heart disease), members can still search out the ways in which cancer affects their constituents directly. In this sense, cancer becomes a local policy issue instead of a national one. As we are about to see, cancer becomes local through the locations of hospitals and the amount of federal funding available to them or through local clusters of severe cancers. Cancer becomes local when universities and medical schools in a member's district are eligible for grant funding through the National Cancer Institute or the National Institutes of Health. Cancer becomes local when interest groups are successful at publicizing the issue to constituents, whether it's through advertisements, word of mouth, or a 5K fundraising event. In any case, not simply cancer, members are apt to look for the local benefit to their support for an issue, because at the end of the day, if the entire nation cares about something but not their district, that will do nothing for their reelection efforts.

This chapter examines how the Congress examines and considers cancer policy. Like the president, the Congress is quite susceptible, if not more so, to the political contours of cancer, particularly at the local level. They are also more vulnerable to economic considerations because of the access that lobbyists and interest groups have to members. But surprisingly, they are quite involved in evaluating the science of cancer and the medical advice of different academic bodies and societies, this from a group that is more often composed of lawyers than doctors and scientists. This chapter begins, like the previous one, with a broad overview, first of powers and motivations, and second of patterns, in this case the amount and types of hearings that the Congress has held in the postwar era. Following this analysis, we will turn more specifically to the politics, the social aspects, the scientific considerations, and the economic impacts affecting members of Congress when it comes to cancer policy.

An Overview of the Congress

Many Americans often feel like they have a good grasp of what the Congress is and what it does; unfortunately, time and time again, polls looking at the political knowledge of those everyday Americans find just the opposite. Although a comprehensive overview of the Congress is best left to other texts or classes, we will briefly discuss some of the more relevant concepts about Congress that are intrinsic to understanding how they behave with regard to cancer policy. First, to the extent to which the president was the only nationally elected figure, members of Congress are almost hyperlocal. Representatives in the House represent small portions of states called districts, whereas members of the Senate represent entire states. Because of this, national issues don't typically appeal to members of Congress (MCs), particularly MCs in the House. Why would this be the natural inclination of MCs? Shouldn't we want a Congress that can look at national issues and think about them in a considered and thoughtful way? While this may be ideal, unfortunately, the gritty reality is that MCs are far more interested in one thing: reelection.

In his 1974 political science classic, David Mayhew posited one simple hypothesis that he believed guided representative behavior more than anything else. His idea was that politicians are single-minded seekers of reelection, "It has to be the *proximate* goal of everyone, the goal that must be achieved over and over if other ends are to be entertained."[1] In order to be elected or reelected, then, representatives must please those who will potentially vote for them, the citizens in their district or state. It makes no sense to deal with national trends, as they cannot control them.[2] Instead, MCs focus on what they can do to please their voters and focus on local interests and issues. A recent example of just how important pleasing local voters can be is the case of former Republican House Majority Leader Eric Cantor. Running for reelection in 2014 in what was thought to be a "safe" district, Cantor lost in the primary to a challenger who spent far less money than he. In the wake of such an upset, it became apparent that the voters punished Cantor for not paying enough attention to their issues and too much attention to national and Republican Party concerns.

We often see these local motivations play out in the types of activities MCs undertake in Congress. The most significant activity that we know the Congress is *supposed* to do is write and pass laws. Being the *legislative* branch, the Constitution endows Congress with the ability to actually create the laws and policies under which this country is to be run. And while legislative productivity has ebbed and flowed over the years, in the past decade, legislative productivity has fallen to historically low levels. Reasons for this variously include high levels of polarization and extreme cases of partisan gerrymandering but also the elimination of line items in bills that would extend pork barrel benefits to various MCs. Inclusion of these line items was usually intended to convince significant MCs to vote for a bill; if everyone had a local interest in a bill being passed, it would be more likely to do so. However, with Republican Party policy aimed at eliminating such inducements, legislating has become even harder to achieve nowadays.

These aren't the only reasons that legislating is difficult. Even in periods of unified party control or low party polarization, writing laws is perhaps the most difficult and time-consuming task of the Congress. Policies can be quite complicated with many different interested stakeholders from across the country. Negotiations might need to be conducted between the Congress and the president, who must ultimately sign the bill in order for it to become law. Members must also figure out how they will pay for their legislation. And while the outcome of legislating is often very public, the nitty-gritty, behind-the-scenes negotiating, writing, and hardballing often goes unseen by the people who mean the most to members—their voters.

It's not hard to understand, then, why the rate at which bills have been written and passed has dropped off in recent years. However, there are other activities which MCs often participate in that can mean just as much as legislating. One such activity is the function of Congress commonly known as oversight, or the ability to ensure that the government is operating properly and as intended. The usual form that oversight takes is the investigation of government activities and the calling of congressional hearings where MCs can listen to testimony from those in and outside of government about policy or the goings-on in government. Committee hearings can be called by one person and one person only, the committee chair, thereby eliminating the need to corral the 535 cats in the House and Senate to try to pass a law. Hearings and investigations can be tailored to the interests of particular members and publicized to interested audiences. MCs have the opportunity to speak with, criticize, and cajole relevant bureaucracies. And while hearings can be productive, today they have become little more than publicized grandstanding for many members.

Hearings and investigations can be signals to important constituencies that their concerns and voices are being heard, particularly when the chances of passing legislation are low or there's nothing legislation could do about it. MCs can claim to have done *something* about constituent issues in merely holding one and can draw even greater attention to themselves when the hearings are held outside of Washington, D.C., and in their actual communities. More so than legislation, hearings are a way for MCs to tell their constituents "I hear you and I'm doing the best I can" even if that is followed up with "It's the intransigent other party that's keeping me from doing more."

A final task that we expect Congress to complete is that of budgeting. Nothing gets done in government if no money is appropriated to do so. While this has traditionally been accomplished on an annual basis, in recent years this, too, has become a contested area of activity. All of the factors that contribute to making legislating so difficult have also affected budgeting along with the economic recession, increased calls for a balanced budget, and growing entitlement costs. As such, instead of passing formal budgets on a yearly basis, Congress has resorted to passing what are called "continuing resolutions," keeping government running at the same dollar level as the last passed budget.

In any case, today's Congress is hampered by hyperpartisanship and divided government. It is more difficult than ever for Congress to do anything, yet this is exactly what the founding fathers wished to achieve. They wanted to make it difficult for the Congress to act so that instead of acting too quickly, they could take their time and fully consider the consequences of their actions. However, it is certainly a fine line between careful consideration and obstinate stubbornness.

The Congress and Cancer

To get a look at how the Congress has acted toward cancer policy in the postwar era, we can easily examine the number and types of hearings that members have called. Although it's important to remember that many of these may be symbolic and have little or no actual significance, the holding of a hearing means that at least one member of Congress has concerns about the given policy. For this purpose, we searched through congressional hearings from 1945–2015 looking for hearings that were either significantly or solely focused on cancer and its attendant issues. In this time period, there were a total of 217 congressional hearings on cancer at an average of three per year. Figure 5.1 displays the frequency of cancer hearings held by the House and the Senate.

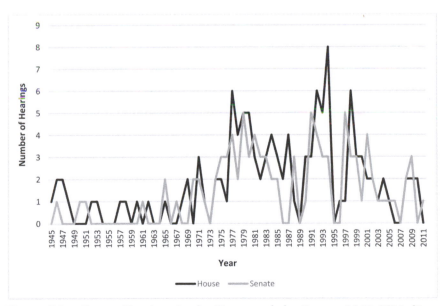

Figure 5.1 Cancer Hearings in the House and the Senate, 1945–2011 (Pro-Quest Congressional Hearings Database)

   While House and Senate hearings have generally tracked similarly, it is
obvious in Figure 5.1 that there are particular periods in which cancer
hearings were held more frequently, specifically the 1970s and 1980s and
then the mid-to-late 1990s. One other way in which we can examine this
data is on the *type* of hearing that was being held, either policy or oversight.
The difference between policy and oversight is very simple; policy hearings
are those hearings in which a committee and its members are considering potential legislation and gathering information on what type of policy to
possibly deploy. Oversight hearings are those that review already enacted
policies or legislation or examine the way in which bureaucracies are
operating. In determining which hearings are policy oriented or oversight
oriented we can also see what types of issues MCs are interested in and
responding to at different points in time.

   Figure 5.2 presents the frequency of policy and oversight related hearings. What is apparent from this data is that although policy hearings still
take place, following the 1971 passage of the National Cancer Act and the
inauguration of Nixon's war on cancer, oversight-related hearings dominated the congressional agenda. This signifies that the role of policy ini-
tiator in some ways had been passed or ceded to the president, whereas in
the years prior, policy had been a congressionally dominated area.

   For ease of analysis, we can break up the pattern of cancer hearings into
four different eras, 1945–1965, 1965–1990, 1990–2011, and 2011–present.

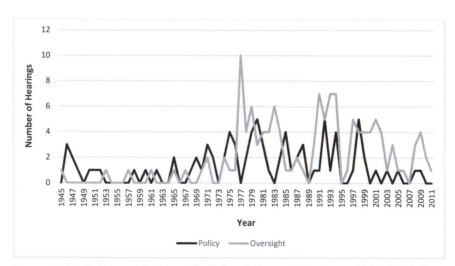

Figure 5.2   Policy- and Oversight-Related Cancer Hearings, 1945–2011 (Pro-
Quest Congressional Hearings Database)

1945–1965

In the first 20 years after World War II, interest in cancer in Congress remained low. At most, three total hearings were held, and most of these were of a general and local nature. In fact, members of Congress apparently knew very little about the National Cancer Institute or any of its programs if a statement from a 1945 hearing is any indication. In a hearing on Aid to the Physically Handicapped (this particular hearing focusing on cancer), Representative Ellis Patterson of California questioned Dr. R.R. Spencer, then head of the NCI. Following Dr. Spencer's opening statement, Representative Patterson engaged in a telling line of questioning, first asking Dr. Spencer where the NCI is located and if it is run "entirely with Federal funds." Some questions later, Representative Patterson asked, "Do you aid in the erection of new institutions or hospitals for cancer in particular? We are trying to start a new hospital in [sic] Los Angeles area. In what way can your institute give assistance?"[3] This interchange is indicative of two things: one, how little Patterson, and presumably other members of the House, knew about the NCI and its activities, and two, the dominance of local concerns which would lead to his later admonition to Dr. Spencer that, "I would like to see you do something on the Pacific coast. At times I think we are so far away the Government sometimes forgets that we exist. We need to provide for our growing population, and we are isolated from the activities of the Government to a considerable extent."[4]

While the frequency of hearings is low, two other things can be noted about this period. One, the House tended to hold hearings more frequently than the Senate, although this certainly isn't saying too much. Second, the hearings that were held tended to be policy related in nature. For example, in 1946, the House held hearings on legislation that would have called for a meeting of the world's cancer experts to consider treatment and cures for cancer. This represents a very early call for not only a cure but also a concerted government-backed effort at pursuing it. Similarly, in 1947, further legislation was considered that proposed to find a cure for cancer along with other diseases such as polio, as well as the establishment of a national cancer research commission. Notably, in the hearing on proposal for a cancer research committee, a letter from then presidential science advisor Vannevar Bush was included in the committee record which downplayed the need for such a group, reflecting presidential noninterest in the move.

Even though attention toward cancer was limited overall, the focused policy consideration coming so shortly after the end of World War II not only demonstrates an interest in the House in particular to take on cancer as a disease, but an increasing concern about the growing prevalence of cancer as a cause of death and the attendant media attention. With the House in particular focused on local aspects of cancer policy, the patterns demonstrated in Figures 5.1 and 5.2 are to be expected given the powers and motivations of MCs.

1965–1990

In many ways, this period is the heart of cancer's consideration in Congress. Additionally, congressional activity tracks well against presidential activity, demonstrating the confluence of two major political actors and their ability to actually achieve a policy output, the National Cancer Act. Throughout the 1960s, Figure 5.1 shows a general build-up in the frequency of hearings, going from one or two a year to five in 1971. This trend is again consistent with what we see with presidential statements, but it is also reflective of the president's policy agenda as well. In a 1965 hearing in the House of Representatives on regional medical complexes for heart disease, cancer, and other diseases, the committee chair, Oren Harris stated, "This morning the committee initiates hearings on HR 3140 [a proposal to establish such medical centers], a bill which I introduced earlier in this session at the request of the President. It is one of the top proposals on the administration's program."[5] This is clear evidence that the Congress was acting not only on its own initiative but on the urging of President Johnson, who was in turn being lobbied extensively by Mary Lasker and the ACS.

Additionally, in this build-up of hearings, both the House and Senate track approximately the same in their frequency, with Senate activity in particular picking up in the mid-to-late 1960s. Given all of the political and global turmoil of that time period, the fact that the Congress and especially the president were able to make room on their agendas for such a topic as cancer demonstrates just how far the policy had come in the postwar years. And these hearings, further, were not simply responding to the goings-on in government, overseeing the actions of cancer programs already in place. Figure 5.2 clearly shows that the types of hearings that were being held were policy oriented, meaning MCs were focusing their efforts on crafting responses to the growing cancer epidemic. These policy-type hearings would continue well into the 1970s, even after the passage of the National Cancer Act, thereby showing a sustained interest not only in crafting a response but a well-reasoned response.

The crux of the 1965–1990 era comes, obviously, with Nixon's war on cancer proposal and the passage of the National Cancer Act in 1971. Immediately following this, there is an exceptional increase in the frequency of hearings on cancer, with a total of 10 hearings in 1977, 6 alone in the House of Representatives. Many of these hearings reflect not only the newly found war on cancer, but other policy concerns of the decade such as environmental issues. For example, a report by the Government Accountability Office (a nonpartisan investigatory agency for the Congress) found that federal efforts to protect the public from carcinogenic chemicals were highly inadequate.[6] This same report specifically faulted the director of the National Cancer Institute for not doing more to promulgate government-wide standards and policies for regulating such chemicals. This focus not only reflects the intense congressional interest around cancer in this time period, but also an awareness of the public criticism that the NCI in particular was not devoting enough energy and dollars into investigations of environmentally based cancers.

After rising to 10 hearings in 1977, the rate at which hearings were held begins to drop off and their focus changes. Instead of focusing primarily on policy-related issues, both the House and the Senate begin to shift their attention to issues of oversight connected not just with the National Cancer Act but also with the NCI in particular. Another congressional concern also begins to make its appearance, that of local interest. One such example is a 1980 House hearing on community-based cancer control programs. Meeting outside of Washington, D.C., in Mineola, New York, Representative Doug Walgren said in his opening statement,

> Today we intend to focus on the community-based cancer control programs. Last year the Congress directed that certain program dollars, namely, $17 million, be placed in the national toxicology program for carcinogenesis testing. This is out of a budget of approximately $70 million for cancer control activities. At the same time, Congress was clear in indicating its intent that it did not intend to have the community cancer program activities cut.
>
> We are therefore concerned to learn whether the issues relating to local community cancer programs and the decisions made by the National Cancer Institute concerning the withdrawal of support for programs such as the Long Island Cancer Center are because of a lack of funds, because of a transfer of funds from the control program to other activities deemed more important, or because of inadequate performances of such programs.[7]

This very local concern is representative and reflective of the types of concerns and motivations that members of Congress, and in particular members in the House of Representatives have; they want to ensure that not only are they "bringing home the bacon" but they are seen as advocating for their communities, especially when they can bring those committee hearings directly into the community.

What is particularly intriguing about the pattern of hearings throughout the 1980s is that despite the fact that for Ronald Reagan cancer ranked very low on the policy agenda, cancer remained a stalwart issue for members of Congress. Hearing topics throughout the decade responded to items as varied as local cancer clusters to media and public criticism of the NCI, as well as the standards by which the NCI operated their drug trials. In this sense, even though no new policy was promulgated or adopted, the Congress remained involved in shaping cancer policy through its oversight function.

1990–2011

In examining Figure 5.1, the year 1989 serves as an appropriate endpoint for the previous era of cancer consideration and the beginning of another. No hearings were held in either the House or the Senate in this year, a stunning fact given that for most of the 20 previous years, the Congress did not let a year go by without taking up some aspect of cancer in the United States. It is quite possible that the HIV/AIDS crisis soaked up much of the policy and political attention in that year, particularly since it was the first year of the George H.W. Bush administration. Despite that, moving into the 1990s, we again see a very active period for congressional consideration of cancer.

Unlike the previous era, however, when new policy directions were being considered, written, and enacted, no new major policies were proposed by either president in office in the 1990s, Bush or Clinton. This is again reflected in the types of hearings that were held which were overwhelmingly oversight oriented. The highest point in the entire series actually comes in 1994 and though this might initially make sense given Bill Clinton's pursuit of health care reform the same year, only one of the hearings was geared toward exploring cancer in the context of health care reform or vice versa. Instead, six of the hearings focused on issues surrounding breast cancer and mammography standards and guidelines, including one that looked specifically at breast cancer in northeast Ohio. So instead of a connection to health care reform, Congress was responding to the increased efforts of breast cancer interest groups and efforts at raising public awareness of breast cancer that were all coalescing at about this time.

Following this intense scrutiny of cancer in general and breast cancer in particular in 1994 again followed a year with no hearings whatsoever in 1995. One possible reason for this decline was the newly empowered Republican Revolution in the Congress which found the Republican Party in the majority in both chambers for the first time in decades. With most of its new members pledged to Newt Gingrich's Contract with America and a greater focus on a balanced budget, cancer was temporarily taken off the political agenda.

This did not last long, however, and 1996 brought in another series of mostly oversight-oriented hearings. While hearings continued to focus on breast cancer and its related issues, other hearings delved into specific decisions on chemicals by the EPA or the FDA, as well as a rising awareness of prostate cancer. What is the most interesting, however, about this period is that following 1998, the rate of cancer hearings begins to drop for the next decade, bottoming out with no hearings in the House in 2006 and no hearings in the Senate in 2007. Unlike the 1980s when Reagan's disinterestedness in cancer was not reflected in the amount and types of hearings MCs held, clearly Bush's choice to not focus on cancer was reflected. Of course, like Bush, the Congress also had to deal with the fallout of not only September 11, but of the wars in Iraq and Afghanistan, a Democratic takeover in 2006, and an economy that faced crisis in 2008.

There is a small spike at the end of this era in 2009 and 2010, the years in which Barack Obama's health care reform plans were being created and pursued. But once again, none of these hearings considered the confluence of cancer and health care reform. Instead, they focused more generically on issues in cancer research, the effects of cell phone use, and breast and prostate cancer. In fact, these later hearings were far more general than hearings in previous eras had been; perhaps this was a recognition on the part of MCs that the effect that such hearings would have on the public would be quite negligible if they were dialing down into the details of specific programs or policies and instead wished to make a general public splash.

2011–Present

The final era represents the past few years and finds the Congress holding no hearings on cancer whatsoever. Unfortunately, why this should be the case is not immediately apparent. The rate of cancer incidence has not greatly declined, there have been no magic bullets, and there are still local and regional cancer clusters that would surely be on the minds of MCs. The only major change that this could be attributed to was the 2010 midterm elections. Those elections found Barack Obama and congressional Democrats heavily penalized electorally with Republicans taking over the majority of both chambers. And to further the issue, the newly elected Republicans were more partisan than previously, a reflection of the growing conservative and Tea Party movement. For these newly empowered

Republicans, "Obamacare" was a derogatory term and there were partisan goals to be accomplished. Perhaps the fight against cancer simply fell victim to the partisan and political goals of the new majority.

In looking at the types of hearings that were held post-2011, many of them do seem to be organized around a partisan and critical theme. Hearings like "High Prices, Low Transparency: The Bitter Pill of Health Care Costs"[8] or "The Roll Out of HealthCare.gov: The Limitations of Big Government"[9] were clearly designed to exploit political issues and extract a political cost. In such an environment, it is not surprising that an issue such as cancer, which does not necessarily lend itself to such fighting, would pay a heavy burden in its reduction of attention.

Summary

This broad overview of congressional action with regard to cancer in the amount and types of hearings that members have held demonstrated three things. First, they do rise and fall somewhat cyclically based on public awareness, interest group activity, and policy action. Congressional attention to cancer is not at all consistent in its amount or its focus. This almost ADD-like attention to cancer and its various policy components does not lend itself to careful consideration of the policy issues. Instead— item two—cancer hearings are susceptible to the politics of the times; when other policy issues crowd the agenda, cancer is easily moved further down the totem pole. Unfortunately, it is not an area in which sustained attention is given to it, for better or for worse. Finally, when and how members of Congress pay attention to cancer is contingent on their own political motivations and reelection-oriented behavior. They are responsive to public criticism and awareness and involved in local and regional issues surrounding cancer. In this sense, this could contribute to the disjointed efforts at crafting a coherent cancer policy as the state and local issues overwhelm MCs in crafting any piece of legislation.

We now turn to look at these patterns through a political, social, scientific, and economic lens.

The Political and Social Elements of Cancer in Congress

Throughout this book, we have generally considered political and social variables separately; however, in this case, there is a very thin line between political and media attention to cancer that the Congress reacts to and the social pressure they experience. Before delving into that arena, in addition to the local concern that we have already discussed, two other political factors appear to be at play with Congress: budgeting and bureaucratic actions. First, with regard to the actions of the various bureaucracies involved in making and enforcing cancer policy, beginning in the 1970s, Congress was much more likely to respond with hearings to decisions or actions that were considered controversial or politically unpalatable. For example, a number of hearings in the 1970s dealt with EPA and FDA actions on chemicals like vinyl chloride and diethylstilbestrol. More significantly, a series of hearings were held in the wake of the FDA's proposal to ban the artificial sweetener saccharin; between 1977 and 1979, there were a total of six hearings on saccharin alone. Other chemicals that would come in for congressional review included nitrites, formaldehyde, ethylene dibromide, phosphate slag, and the fire retardant tris.

In looking at the hearings on saccharin in particular, members of Congress repeatedly expressed outrage not only at the decision but the way in which the FDA made and announced it. In his opening statement to the first oversight hearing on the saccharin ban, Senator Edward Kennedy stated:

> No regulatory action in recent memory has so angered the American people as the decision by the Food and Drug Administration to begin the process of removing saccharin from the market. The decision would have been controversial under any circumstances, but was made more offensive by the inept manner in which the decision was made. Initially, when it counted, the FDA made no effort at public education. There was no attempt to give a complete picture of the scientific evidence upon which the decision was based. FDA officials pictured themselves originally as the helpless victims of a restrictive law that required the removal of a substance, which, when force fed to rats in overwhelming quantities, caused an increase in the incidence of cancer.[10]

What is even more stunning about this criticism is the person who was making it: arch-Democrat Edward Kennedy. Particularly in the late 1970s under the Carter administration, the regulatory atmosphere was far more conducive to bureaucratic actors making such decisions and taking such actions. The fact that the FDA was suddenly facing criticism from those who had previously championed the effort (and from one who would later go on to suffer a vicious form of brain cancer) must have been surprising.

The Democratic criticism of the saccharin ban is not limited to this one case. In fact, throughout the 1970s and 1980s, the very period in which the Congress questioned bureaucratic decisions on a wide variety of chemicals, the institution was largely Democratic. Following the Republican takeover of Congress in 1994, there were actually no hearings specifically looking at these regulatory actions. We thus have a conundrum; the party that we have found to be more proactive and favorably disposed toward regulations is also the same party that has tended to ask the most questions about those regulations. Perhaps this is simply a case of more regulatory decisions to question; when more regulations are promulgated, some might emerge that are more controversial than would be created under Republican Party control. In any case, this fact demonstrates that perhaps Democrats are not willing to go along with all regulatory actions and are willing to keep a closer eye on those decisions.

A second political element which has yet to be addressed in this chapter is that of budgeting. Because this is an annual process, it allows members of Congress a routine and regular means through which to oversee cancer policy and make any necessary changes. It should be noted that no budgetary hearings were included in the tally that has been used thus far because there were never any budget hearings that focused *specifically* on the NCI. What is usually the case is that the activities and operations of the NCI get lumped in with the Department of Health and Human Services, the National Institutes of Health, and other related program areas. However, some things can be said about budgeting for cancer and congressional hearings. First, it is indicative of the amount of attention that the Congress pays toward the NCI that they did not hold hearings specifically on the agency; either they did not feel the program significant enough to do so or the NCI simply isn't a contentious or difficult issue to consider when it comes to budgeting.

And although we will discuss a special case of appropriations hearings on cancer later that has a social tinge to it, we should not forget that in any case, the analysis of Chapter 2 helps to inform our discussion here. The mixed findings on the role of party and the noninfluence of election years says a lot about the politics that are *not* involved in cancer policy; we don't see much of a concern with budgeting, but we do see a great interest in local issues.

This is where the political begins to meld into the social, and there are two topics to be covered here. First, there have been some hearings about cancer within the Senate Appropriations Committee: in 1997 there were three, one each in 1998, 2002, 2005, and 2006, and two each in 1999, 2001, and 2009. Why and in what context have these hearings been held? The topics of the hearings ranged broadly from breast cancer to prostate cancer to blood cancer but they all generally focused on the efforts of the NIH and the National Institute of Medicine's efforts toward these diseases. But the other common thread that runs through these hearings is who was calling them: first Senator Arlen Specter and then Senator Tom Harkin.

In the opening to one such hearing in 1998, Senator Specter details the efforts that he and Senator Harkin had been making to increase funding for scientific research at the NIH, demonstrating that these congressional hearings were being used to pursue such a goal. But for Specter, the driving force was even more personal; in the same opening, Specter details the cases of four individuals close to him who had experienced or were experiencing cancer. He stated, "I look at my three grandchildren and I look at my own PSA score and I see the people who are here today, prostate cancer survivors, and say that we ought to be funding every last research grant which is meritorious. We can afford to do it and we cannot afford not to do it."[11] Arlen Specter would go on to be diagnosed with Hodgkin's lymphoma in 2005 and remained in the Senate while undergoing chemotherapy. He would die from non-Hodgkin's lymphoma in 2012.

This personal connection to cancer is something that falls under the realm of social elements; like the presidents we discussed in the previous chapter, Senator Specter appeared deeply affected by the curse of cancer. Surrounded by people who were experiencing it and concerned about his own health, he had a personal motivation to increase funding and encourage greater research into a cure for cancer. Undoubtedly, a number of representatives and senators have had similar experiences or experienced cancer themselves. Being a far larger institution than the presidency (an office of one), the chances are simply higher that more people will be personally affected by the disease. Perhaps this is why cancer funding is somewhat easy to come by; no one is going to want to vote down a cancer research bill when it could theoretically benefit not only their constituents and their families but also themselves. In short, being pro-cancer is good politics.

A second social-political element to be discussed is the role of the media and its relationship to public attention. To this point, we have not really had to specify the line between what is media driven and what is socially driven; in reality, this line is quite hard to find. Is it public attention that drives media coverage or vice versa? While we romanticize the ideal that the media is a reflection of what the public is interested in and excited about, that is hardly the reality. The reality is that more often than not, the choices of the media and its newsmakers and news writers serve to set the agenda for not only the public but the political world as well. In this case, we might view media attention as the political and public awareness as the social. That being said, this is a perfect example of how these two spheres can overlap and interact in a way that makes categorization hard.

The response to media attention is only natural when one thinks back to our discussion of presidential politics. Even the Congress must appear to respond to issues, particularly when they are brought to the light of public awareness. One primary example of this phenomenon was a series of hearings in 1981 that specifically responded to a series of articles in *The Washington Post* criticizing the state of the NCI's drug program. In his opening statement, Representative Henry Waxman specifically referenced these articles and argued that "[t]he criticism has done great injury to the [National Cancer] Institute's public credibility and cause many to question the wisdom of the Congress [sic] traditional hands-off support."[12] Not content with merely speaking about the *Post* articles, the articles themselves were even inserted into the hearing record, reinforcing the media-driven nature of the hearing.

One way to examine this hearing–media link is to examine the number of cancer articles published in *The New York Times*, a set of data we used in Chapter 2 compared to the number of hearings per year. This graph is shown in Figure 5.3; Although the data is clearly on different scales, you can see an uptick in hearings with media attention to cancer rises, particularly in and around 1994. This is the same year when hearings on breast cancer dominated despite the concern with health care. For further evidence of this correlation, we can look to the Pearson correlation value, which is significant at 0.416, indicating a positive and strong relationship.

That the media was driving public awareness in 1981 seems to be the case; the issues surrounding drug therapy and trials are often difficult to

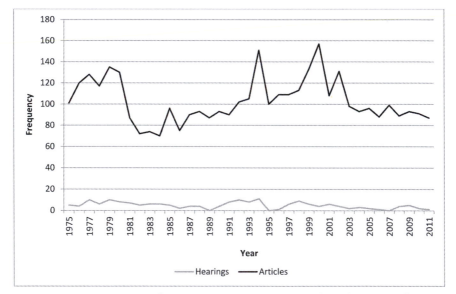

Figure 5.3 Frequency of Cancer Hearings Compared with *New York Times* Cancer Articles, 1975–2011

understand and digest, hardly the type of issue that gets spontaneously picked up for public consumption. However, the other spike in this data in 1994 is most likely a case of social awareness driving the press coverage. During this period in particular, the breast cancer movement was riding a high wave of participation and knowledge; not only could everyone have a personal connection to it, but various interest groups had succeeded in coalescing and cooperating in their promotion efforts, and there were a series of new scientific developments related to breast cancer.[13] Breast cancer was and remains a disease that can strike at the heart of every family; everyone has *at least* a mother and grandmothers and even men could suffer from it. Historically, there were horrendously terrible treatment options available. The radical mastectomy pioneered in the early 20th century not only removed the affected breast tissue but much of the surrounding tissue, lymph nodes, and even bone leaving many women deeply disfigured.

Despite this history, the early 1990s were a period of hope for breast cancer patients; studies on tamoxifen as both a treatment and preventative measure were ongoing and their results astounding. The discovery of the BRCA1 and BRCA2 genes that increased a woman's chances of getting breast cancer had just been discovered and a diagnostic test fashioned in 1994. This combination of social and scientific forces would make headline news, driving not only coverage in the media but an uptick in the hearings held in Congress.

Social forces have not ceased to play a role in driving the actions of Congress. Moving into the 21st century, Congress has held hearings on other specific cancers such as cervical cancer, prostate cancer, and leukemia. Most likely, this has been driven by increasing interest group involvement in cancer. Following on the success of the breast cancer movement, patients and their families suffering with other types of cancers have often tried to replicate the success that breast cancer has had. We can see this not only in the pink that professional sports teams will often wear to promote breast cancer awareness, but also more recently the light blue that Major League Baseball in particular has adopted around Father's Day to promote prostate cancer research.

It is interesting, though, how in dealing with the Congress this is the first time we have confronted the intermingling of political and social forces. This simply demonstrates how much more vulnerable but open the Congress is to the rest of society as the people's representatives. They must face reelection on an unrelenting basis. They are accountable to the people who put them in office. Whereas the bureaucracies are quite insulated from social movements and the president less so, the Congress is quite exposed to the whims and social movements of the American public, something the American founding fathers realized early on. This is not a bad thing; we expect our legislators to be open to the concerns of their voters and mirror the issues that they find most important.

Science in the Congress: Questioning Authority

For a body of elected officials that only rarely contains a scientist, medical doctor, or other type of researcher, if you judge by the types of hearings that have been held, members of Congress are very interested and involved in the science of cancer. Although they are not necessarily involved in the detailed work involved in setting up a clinical trial or preparing results and interpreting them, they have historically been attentive to just those activities. In examining the pattern of congressional hearings, two major scientific areas have been questioned: the practice of clinical trials and the release of advice from medical bodies and associations.

As we have discussed before, despite its apparent objectivity and sheen of neutrality, science and the state of knowledge is indeed a very political thing. Many of the hearings that have questioned the science of cancer reflect a statement made by Representative John Dingell in a hearing on a study of formaldehyde in 1986: "However, I am concerned about the NCI's recently concluded formaldehyde study, which I feel raises serious questions about possible dangerous new trends in *occupational cancer epidemiological research* at NCI."[14] Representative Dingell was not questioning the results of the study so much as the pattern of the study itself. For the formaldehyde study in particular, Dingell and his colleagues were questioning the absence of input from interested stakeholders in labor and other federal agencies.

This hearing was not abnormal for the period; the decade of the 1980s saw a significant uptick in the frequency with which members of Congress questioned the state of clinical trials within the NCI. In a 1981 hearing focused on oversight of the NCI, Senator Paula Hawkins argued that the NCI is inflicted by the cancers "of inaction, confusion, indecision, frustration, delay, and failure to communicate."[15] Specifically, Senator Hawkins was concerned about the state of clinical trials at the NCI and its relationship with the FDA, which was discussed in Chapter 2. Finding multiple instances of unregulated or poorly organized clinical trials, the committee severely criticized the NCI for its lack of control over its scientists and poor record keeping.

Following up on these concerns a year and a half later, Senator Hawkins held another hearing questioning how safe the drugs that had been given in clinical trials were. Reflecting back on the findings of her first hearing,

Hawkins reported that a Government Accountability Office (GAO) task force examining clinical trials between 1975 and 1980 found that whereas the NCI reported that 9.5 percent of patients responded to treatments in phase I trials, the more likely figure was that less than 5 percent of patients benefitted.[16] The concerns of Senator Hawkins echo those of the FDA in providing clearly toxic treatments to cancer patients, knowing that only a few would find any benefit. What the senators were questioning was the practice of clinical trials and the judgment of doctors and medical professionals to treat patients. In fact, Senator Hawkins herself states that because "we have not yet devised a mechanism to oversee the actual interaction of the doctor with the patient, the informed consent form itself assumes great importance."[17] While I doubt that Senator Hawkins was actually calling for government intervention into the doctor–patient relationship, the inference is that the NCI at the very least should be informing patients more fully of their options.

Other hearings questioning the science of cancer in the 1980s included two hearings on the implications of oncogene research and cancer survival rates. Mirroring a more societal concern about whether the war on cancer was succeeding and a scientific debate on the right types of statistics to be used, Congress waded into the battle itself in 1987. After requesting a study of cancer survival and incidence rates, Representative Henry Waxman noted that the "GAO concluded that even the basic statistics used to describe survival need attention and clarification."[18] Even the GAO's study of statistics needed defending from critics of the war on cancer; the GAO's representative Eleanor Chelimsky, who testified at the hearing, specifically argued against the notion that the report was "somehow biased against positive findings" and was "subjective or opinion-based."[19] Even the congressionally commissioned study examining the statistics of cancer survival and incidence had to battle perceived notions of bad methodology and subjective attitudes.

Congressional concern with science continued into the 1990s where hearings were held on the "Scientific and Technical Bases for Radon Policy"[20] and the linear no-threshold model of low-dose radiation. The hearing on the science of radon is particularly intriguing for the statement of the committee chair, Senator J. Bennett Johnston, recognizing the uncertainty of science and specifically questioning whether "the views and data of scientists have not been faithfully transmitted and have not been accompanied by the necessary caveats when presented to policymakers in the Congress. In fact, the existing record on this topic has a recurring pattern of snappy sound bites and distorted facts that do not stand up to close scrutiny when one looks for the supporting data."[21]

On the one hand, although it is somewhat comforting to know that members of Congress are questioning the science and the facts that are being given to them in order to make policy, on the other hand, it is disconcerting to know that in many cases they are already skeptical of the science being handed to them, even from nonpartisan agencies like the GAO. Surely, good oversight of bureaucratic programs requires an examination of the science supporting the policy and its various activities, but these examples continue to document the political and social nature of knowledge itself. And when this is done potentially by nonscientists, the understanding and interpretation of scientific data can become quite dangerous.

What is potentially even more dangerous is the congressional questioning of medical advice given by professional bodies and even government agencies. Imagine, men and women across the country looking to the advice of their health professionals only to have it questioned by one of the most powerful bodies in the United States. The most prominent example of this phenomenon has to do with mammography and the guidelines that have been issued for when women should begin to be screened for breast cancer via mammograms. Proponents of more aggressive annual checks on a yearly basis argue that early detection is vital to saving lives and catching cancer at an earlier stage. However, opponents note that there is a high chance of false-positive test results leading to unnecessary fear, anxiety, and biopsies.

The discussion around mammography guidelines first erupted in 1994 when the NCI overruled an advisory body on recommendations for screening for women age 40–49. The advisory board voted to recommend annual screening for women beginning at age 40; however, the NCI did not go along with the recommendation. In his opening statement, the committee chair, Representative Edolphus Towns, was incensed at the NCI's actions, criticizing not only the decision but the process through which the decision had been made. This included the questioning of the scientific studies that were used in the decision itself. After stating that the NCI had used eight randomized clinical trials (the gold standard for hypothesis testing), Representative Towns states,

> CI's reliance solely on these eight randomized clinical trials to set the mammography guidelines for millions of women in this country remains questionable. Of these eight trials, only 30 percent of the participants were in the 40 to 49 age group. Further, only one trial was conducted on American women, and that was the oldest trial in the group with the oldest technology.[22]

This questioning of scientific methodology is a classic play on scientific criticism that was discussed in both Chapters 2 and 3. Towns concludes that perhaps the change in guidance from the NCI stems from change in personnel that "has facilitated academics and MDs with little medical experience with breast cancer patients to set in motion an agenda to impose science over medicine and change the guidelines."[23]

In a later iteration of these concerns, a hearing in the Senate in 2002 continued to question the science behind mammography guidelines. Senator Barbara Mikulski identified this concern, saying, "I understand dissent in the scientific community and differences of opinion about particular studies, but this conflict is exasperating . . . In the absence of clarity, I'm concerned that these conflicting studies give an excuse to insurance companies to stop paying for mammograms."[24] Despite all of the *sturm und drang* centered on the mammography controversy, in the many years since mammography recommendations have been handed down, we have come no further on specifically nailing down when women with no family or personal history of breast cancer should begin to receive annual mammograms. As of 2016, the American Cancer Society recommends annual screening beginning at age 45, whereas the American College of Obstetricians and Gynecologists says age 40, and the U.S. Preventative Services Task Force says age 50.

It is actually rather ironic that over time the Congress has found itself mired not just in the politics of breast cancer but in the politics of screening for breast cancer. While politicians nominally cite the high costs socially, economically, and personally of breast cancer, the fact that breast cancer is intimately connected to women's health and sexuality makes their concern even more unusual. Others have clearly noted the political concern with intimate women's issues such as abortion and family planning, but this is yet another example of apparently deeply interested (for better or worse) politicians have been in the sexual health of women.

The Economics of Cancer

Members of Congress are very susceptible to economic issues, particularly when they emanate from their own states or districts. Many of their voters will be deciding on whether to vote for them based on the state of the economy; the last thing members will want to do is anger a significant portion of their voter base by damaging the local economy. Although cancer is not immediately linked to any of these economic interests in particular, there are obvious connections that we have discussed. The quantitative model in Chapter 2 uncovered that the number of hospitals in the United States was a factor influencing funding for cancer; think about how this would affect individual states and districts. Much like the congressman from the 1946 hearing discussed earlier, the NCI disburses much of their funds to researchers spread throughout the country. One multimillion-dollar grant can spur not only a series of high-paying jobs but possibly medical and technical breakthroughs that can later be monetized. Further, the presence of highly specialized and trained oncologists and cancer researchers can attract top medical talent, as well as more patients for hospitals and cancer treatment centers.

One example of how the Congress has been influenced by this economic dimension is their concern with patents and drugs developed as a result of government funding and grants. A hearing in 1991 examined agreements between drug manufacturer Bristol-Myers Squibb and various government agencies, including the National Cancer Institute, about drug development. The agreements between the federal government and Bristol-Myers Squibb concerned access to yew trees in the Pacific Northwest that were the only known source of the drug taxol. Chairman Ron Wyden called these agreements "extraordinary because they give near-total control of a life-saving plant species to one drug company, and because they provide exclusive, federally-funded technology to Bristol-Myers Squibb."[25] Although Bristol-Myers would have received a large economic benefit from this agreement, Wyden, a representative of Oregon, was concerned about the environmental and animal impact of such decisions; therefore, it could be said that he was protecting the long-term environmental and even economic interests of his own constituents who would have been affected.

Just two years later, Wyden would again take up the issue of drugs, this time focusing on the pricing of drugs developed through government support. Once again citing the Bristol-Myers controversy, Wyden noted, "The production price paid by the National Cancer Institute for experimental quantities of refined taxol ranged between 60 cents and 90 cents per milligram. Bristol-Myers Squibb has announced it would price the drug at $986 per 3-week treatment cycle or about $4.87 per milligram, a markup of six to eight times NCI's production costs prior to the agreement."[26] In having complete control of the taxol market, Bristol-Myers could have expected up to $800 million in profits.[27] In a rebuttal to Wyden, Zola Horovitz, representing Bristol-Myers, claimed that

[g]reater restrictions on product pricing would reduce incentives for private companies to participate in the CRADA process [the type of agreement the NCI and Bristol-Myers entered into]. Substantial financial incentives are necessary to justify an enormous investment, sometimes measured in hundreds of millions of dollars required for the rapid development of new pharmaceutical products. Few companies are willing or able to make

investments of such magnitude. They want and deserve some assurance that they will have the opportunity to recover these investments and earn a reasonable return.[28]

The crux of the debate, then, is consumer protection from seemingly inflated prices and the economic incentives that companies have to develop drugs. This is a conundrum that continues to plague American public policy as drug companies are often excoriated for their high prices. The economic debate is not simply about the impact on pharmaceutical companies, but also on the costs to consumers.

One other economic connection that has often been considered through congressional hearings is how Medicare policies affect the pricing and type of treatment that is often given to cancer patients. A 1992 GAO study found that Medicare reimbursement policies can strongly influence where patients are treated. "Our review showed that (1) some oncologists have treated cancer patients in hospital inpatient and outpatient settings when, by clinical standards, they could have received treatment in the office," the GAO stated, and "(2) financial factors influence the oncologist's choice of treatment setting."[29] With a booming population of seniors who will be using Medicare treatment in the coming decades, one of the fastest-rising costs will inevitably be cancer treatment; in government decisions about what treatments should be covered and at what rate, Medicare policy can strongly affect cancer treatment.

This has already happened in one other developed country: the United Kingdom. Although the insurance setting is quite different from that of the United States, the problem they face is likely to be faced by U.S. policy makers in short order. Because of the increasing costs of many cancer drugs, in early 2016, the UK's Cancer Drugs Fund decided to stop paying for 45 different cancer indications because of lack of cost-effectiveness data on their use.[30] While this does not change the availability of the drugs to cancer patients in the UK, the issue demonstrates the looming public policy crisis that will exist in the United States as more and more baby boomers come to depend on Medicare for their health care.

Other major players in the economic field include those groups that we will be discussing more fully in the next chapter: interest groups. Because of their more open nature, members of Congress are also widely available to be lobbied, not only by their constituents or business, but by the public interest groups and the hired lobbyists on their payroll. These lobbyists can provide not only information and arguments concerning different public policy issues, but they also provide key resources that members of Congress will need on their road to election and reelection. These resources include, first and foremost, publicity and money, something that major cancer interest groups have been more than willing to provide. In data going back to 2008, the most prolific giver of lobbying-related dollars to members of Congress has been the political arm of the American Cancer Society, the Cancer Action Network. Not only have they thrown thousand-dollar events to the benefit of members, but they have also given directly to campaign reelection funds. Despite their willingness to spend money, the ACS has not spread the love around, so to speak, instead concentrating their efforts on specific members, usually Democrats. The most frequent recipient has been Representative Rosa DeLauro, a survivor of ovarian cancer and proponent of cancer-related issues. This fact is reflective of the trend that interest groups usually give their resources to people who are already likely to be with them in the first place, instead of as enticements to be favorably disposed toward their issues.

The National Breast Cancer Coalition has been the second most active interest group in providing resources to members of Congress. Their main activity has been to hold a large event annually to recognize prominent members of both parties and both chambers, recognizing them for their work on breast cancer issues. Outside of these receptions, campaign donations have been directed exclusively at Democrats, including campaigns for Hillary Clinton in 2008 and 2015.

In looking at an overall picture of congressional hearing activity, there are not many other hearings that specifically address an economic link to cancer. The hearings that members have held, however, have generally included representatives from interest groups like the American Cancer Society as well as industry representatives like the Bristol-Myers Squibb executive discussed earlier. This ensures that the economic interests of the various stakeholders are brought to the table. Of course, the difficult thing about examining interest group impact is that it is near impossible to peer behind the closed doors to see where the actual negotiations and bill writing are done. Unless we are in the room where it happens, we cannot specifically link one action to another. This has historically been a limit for political science research looking at the impact of interest groups on public policy.

Conclusion

We shouldn't be surprised that members of Congress are similar to us; after all, we expect them to be our representatives to the federal government. In facing cancer, we don't necessarily think about the economic impacts right away; that only hits us when we see how much the drug bill will be.

We don't immediately think about the science of cancer until it affects our treatment or what our doctors recommend. But we do react on a visceral, personal level, wanting to do everything we can to beat back a disease that hits all too many of us. Although we can criticize and cajole Congress all we like, decry their lack of progress or bipartisanship, as characterized by this discussion, they do want to help their constituents. Although the ultimate goal is to better themselves through reelection, if the means is by looking after the issues that are vital to their neighbors, then we, too, can reap the benefit.

CHAPTER SIX

The Cancer Community

One of the most preventable cancers is lung cancer; in fact, according to the American Cancer Society, it is the single most preventable cancer in the world.[1] Every year, more than 220,000 people will be newly diagnosed with lung cancer, and more than 159,000 will die from it. The reason that so many people are affected by lung cancer and the reason that it is so preventable is one and the same: these cases of lung cancer are overwhelmingly caused by the use of tobacco. Tobacco causes up to 87 percent of lung cancers in men and 70 percent of lung cancers in women,[2] and that's not the only type of cancer that tobacco use is associated with. Tobacco users are also at higher risks of throat and mouth cancers, stomach, pancreas, kidney, bladder, uterus, and cervix cancers.

Let's take a moment to imagine not only the number of lives saved but what those lives would mean and contribute to society if tobacco were taken out of the equation. Over a 10-year time period, that would mean more than 1.5 million people still alive (or at least not dead due to tobacco), contributing economically, physically, and emotionally to society. That would be more than 1.5 million families who would not know the tragedy and agony of a loved one suffering through this debilitating disease. So why not ban a substance that is so clearly dangerous and addictive and nearly certain to cause death? It would not be the first time government had stepped in to ban such chemicals; they do it on a regular basis. Why not tobacco?

We know almost intuitively why that type of proposal is a nonstarter—the economic power and political prowess of the tobacco industry. Tobacco has been a part of the American economy since before there was an America; growing tobacco was a staple of early agricultural practices and one of the main exports to Europe. That power has only grown as more and more people have become addicted to the nicotine in the tobacco and due to the growth in tobacco use in the early 20th century. That growth contributed to ever-growing profits and power for the companies growing tobacco and turning it into cigars, cigarettes, chewing tobacco, and more recently e-cigarettes. In 2013, the combined revenues of the six largest tobacco companies in the world was more than $342 billion, more than enough to secure for these companies a say in local and national politics.[3] And although the number has been declining, this translates into more than $20 million spent on lobbying in Washington, D.C., alone, with 182 lobbyists.[4] This doesn't even take into account the money that is spent in local and state politics where bans on smoking in public places or the rate of cigarette taxes is decided. And what's more is the economic impact of the tobacco industry itself. Millions of Americans are employed not only farming and processing tobacco, but people are employed by the tobacco firms, the marketing companies, and even those small businesses across America that do a large percentage of their business on tobacco products.

So what is more important to us: the lives of millions of Americans or the billions of dollars in profits for tobacco companies? In all reality, the question is a false dichotomy and can be argued either way. But the point is that the consideration of banning tobacco for health reasons is not a public policy option that is ever mentioned precisely because of the economic impact and power of the tobacco industry.

While economics will not be the sole focus of this chapter, it does have an outsized role to play. This chapter focuses on the interest groups and industry groups that make up what we would call the cancer community. This includes not only the tobacco industry but pharmaceuticals, businesses that are affected by regulations or produce or use carcinogenic chemicals, doctors, nurses, health professionals, hospitals, and the patient community that are all relevant stakeholders in cancer policy in the United States. Obviously, this is a very broad and rich community; it would be nearly impossible to accurately summarize it with justice in the space of a chapter. As such, we will instead focus on a representative actor of three different types of groups that are involved in the cancer community: public interest groups, medical associations, and industry.

The American Cancer Society, as perhaps the longest-operating cancer interest group that has had the biggest impact societally, is an obvious choice as a representative of the interest group community. It is a broad cancer group, not tied specifically to one type of cancer or another, and it has consistently played a role in the politics of cancer since the end of World War II.

As far as medical associations go, there are any number that we could focus on. There is the American Medical Association, perhaps the most well-known medical group in the country, or there are cancer-specific medical associations like the American Society of Clinical Oncology or the Society of Surgical Oncology. Again, for their consistent involvement in politics, including the politics of cancer, we will go broad and detail the activities of the AMA.

Finally, as our discussion of tobacco highlights, many industries are involved with or affected by the politics of cancer. Because the travails of the tobacco industry have been covered extensively elsewhere, we will not rehash the debate. Instead, we will focus on an industry that has the ability to affect just about every cancer patient and their families, the pharmaceutical industry, represented by their major interest group: the Pharmaceutical Research and Manufacturers of America, otherwise known as PhRMA.

In many ways, all three of these actors have been previously discussed in this book in some way. This goes to demonstrate their deep and intricate involvement with cancer policy and politics in the United States. All three are capable political actors that have shown the ability to affect policy outcomes and shape public awareness and opinion on issues relating to cancer and cancer research. And because they are broadly representative of cancer in general, they give us a good handle on cancer politics because delving into more specified types of cancer such as breast cancer or leukemia could leave a skewed impression of the types of politics involved.

The American Cancer Society

Interest groups are strange political creatures. They are important linkages between the government and the voters, but they are not always effective vehicles for policy change. Why might this be the case? One of the most significant problems any interest group, let alone a group like the American Cancer Society, must face is something called the collective action problem. First introduced by Mancur Olsen, collective action problems describe the difficulty that groups have in getting things done, especially when there is the ability for any one person to shirk their responsibility. All of us have faced a scenario like this at one time or another; when trying to get a group to work together and accomplish a task, there is always (or almost always) that one person who knows they will get credit for the solution no matter how little effort they put into it. The collective action problem is this very conundrum blown up on an even larger scale. Think of it this way: if the American Cancer Society funds research that eventually leads to a cure for cancer, that cure would be available to everyone. What is my incentive to participate in a group for which I will get the benefit if I do nothing?

This collective action problem is particularly acute when interest groups are lobbying a government for policy change; their power is enhanced when they have a large number of people behind them, but it is often easier said than done in gathering those numbers. To that end, interest groups like the ACS engage in other activities through which they can make their impact felt. In addition to fundraising activities, they encourage and support research, provide information to the public, and create public awareness campaigns. The ACS as an organization has pursued all of these activities throughout its history.

Today's ACS began as the American Society for the Control of Cancer (ASCC) in New York in 1913. Originally, it was made up primarily of doctors and scientists who wrote reports and carried out public relations campaigns. For much of its early years, its fundraising was outsourced to another organization called the Women's Field Army, which was semi-militant but successful in its ability to raise funds.[5] Beginning in the 1940s, the ASCC came to the attention of Mary Lasker and her husband, Albert, himself an advertising executive. Following a successful Lasker-directed public outreach through *Reader's Digest*, Albert Lasker took a seat on the board of the ASCC and began reforming the organization from the inside out.

Once on the board, Lasker worked to bring in others to the board, but instead of doctors and research scientists, the people who were newly engaged were like him, from the corporate boardroom and executive suites. Little by little, the doctors were relegated to a backseat as the ASCC became the American Cancer Society. With all of these changes, the Women's Field Army was dissolved, and fundraising became a cornerstone activity of the ACS itself. Despite the dominance of business professionals on the board of the ACS, Mary Lasker desired the involvement of a prominent cancer scientist who could serve as the face of oncology and the search for a cure; this face soon became Dr. Sidney Farber of Boston Children's Hospital.[6]

Today, the American Cancer Society is the largest voluntary health organization in the United States with over 2.5 million volunteers.[7] It is organized into 11 geographical divisions with even more local chapters who organize events including Relay for Life. Its mission is "dedicated to eliminating cancer as a major health problem by preventing cancer, saving lives, and diminishing suffering from cancer, through research, education, advocacy, and service."[8] In 2015, they raised over $809 million through public donations and spent over $708 million on cancer services.[9]

Political Elements

As we have discussed previously, the power of the ACS, at least in the mid-20th century, came from its patron, Mary Lasker. Her connections and friendships not only with New York's but Washington, D.C.'s most powerful people put her in a prime position to act as a policy entrepreneur. She was able to influence Lyndon B. Johnson and eventually Richard Nixon to step up government efforts on cancer prevention and research and was a pivotal actor in Nixon's declaration of a war on cancer. Since Lasker, no other single figure has emerged to fill her shoes and follow in the same role. In more recent years, the political power of the ACS has come through its ability to lobby government officials and influence public opinion.

The ACS is a very active lobbying organization and has become more so in the 21st century. From 1998–2004, it spent less than $1 million per year on lobbying expenses at the federal level, beginning in 2004, these numbers began to rise, spiking to almost $10 million in 2006, falling to $3.7 million in 2010, and sat at $5.5 million in 2015.[10] In 2016, the ACS had 20 lobbyists on staff with another lobbyist contracted out to a lobbying firm.[11] Because of disclosure rules, all lobbying organizations must file reports as to the number and type of contacts they have with elected officials, with this data available electronically back to 1998. Table 6.1 tracks the types of issues and the number of reports the ACS has filed on them.

Perhaps the most frequent topic that the ACS lobbies Congress on is the federal budget and appropriations. For example, in 2011 when there were 20 different reports of contact on the budget, the ACS was specifically searching for greater funds for agencies like the NIH and NCI for cancer research and related programs. Other topics ripe for lobbying include the vague category of "health issues" which, in 2015, included health disparities, health care reform, childhood cancer, and the like. What is also apparent from these lobbying contacts is the sustained amount of lobbying on tobacco and tax issues. Although tobacco might not be very surprising, the fact that the ACS, a group concentrated on issues related to cancer, is concerned about taxes is illuminating. On tax-related issues, the ACS reported that specifically, they were lobbying on issues "relating to the tax treatment of nonprofits," something that could have the ability to significantly affect their bottom line if charitable donations were no longer tax exempt or tax exempt to the extent that they currently are.

It is difficult to peer inside the halls of Washington and measure just how effective any given lobbying effort is, but one intriguing case of the

Table 6.1   ACS Lobbying Contacts, 1998–2015

Year	Issues	Number of Reports
1998	Health Issues	5
	Medical Research and Clinical Laboratories	3
	Medicare and Medicaid	3
	Federal Budget and Appropriations	3
	Food Industry	1
	Tobacco	1
1999	Health Issues	6
	Federal Budget and Appropriations	4
	Tobacco	3
	Medical Research and Clinical Laboratories	2
	Medicare and Medicaid	2
	Taxes	2
2000	Federal Budget and Appropriations	4
	Tobacco	4
	Health Issues	2
	Medical Research and Clinical Laboratories	2
	Medicare and Medicaid	2
	Taxes	2
2001	Federal Budget and Appropriations	7
	Tobacco	6
	Health Issues	5
	Medicare and Medicaid	4
	Taxes	4
2002	Federal Budget and Appropriations	6
	Health Issues	4
	Tobacco	3
	Medicare and Medicaid	2
2003	Federal Budget and Appropriations	6
	Health Issues	4
	Medicare and Medicaid	2
	Taxes	2
	Tobacco	2

(continued)

Table 6.1   (*continued*)

Year	Issues	Number of Reports
2004	Federal Budget and Appropriations	9
	Health Issues	7
	Medicare and Medicaid	4
	Tobacco	4
	Taxes	2
2005	Federal Budget and Appropriations	12
	Health Issues	8
	Tobacco	6
	Medicare and Medicaid	3
	Taxes	2
2006	Federal Budget and Appropriations	14
	Health Issues	10
	Tobacco	5
	Medicare and Medicaid	4
	Taxes	3
	Insurance	1
2007	Federal Budget and Appropriations	17
	Health Issues	11
	Tobacco	10
	Medicare and Medicaid	7
	Taxes	4
2008	Health Issues	28
	Federal Budget and Appropriations	20
	Tobacco	17
	Medicare and Medicaid	12
	Taxes	4
2009	Health Issues	25
	Federal Budget and Appropriations	19
	Tobacco	14
	Medicare and Medicaid	10
	Taxes	6

(*continued*)

Table 6.1   (*continued*)

Year	Issues	Number of Reports
2010	Health Issues	23
	Federal Budget and Appropriations	22
	Tobacco	11
	Medicare and Medicaid	11
	Taxes	4
2011	Federal Budget and Appropriations	20
	Health Issues	16
	Medicare and Medicaid	10
	Tobacco	8
	Taxes	4
2012	Health Issues	17
	Federal Budget and Appropriations	14
	Medicare and Medicaid	7
	Tobacco	6
	Taxes	4
2013	Health Issues	12
	Federal Budget and Appropriations	7
	Medicare and Medicaid	4
	Taxes	4
	Tobacco	4
	Trade	4
2014	Federal Budget and Appropriations	8
	Taxes	7
	Tobacco	4
	Trade	4
	Health Issues	4
	Medicare and Medicaid	4
2015	Federal Budget and Appropriations	8
	Health Issues	4
	Medicare and Medicaid	4
	Taxes	4
	Tobacco	4
	Trade	1

Source: Center for Responsive Politics, http://www.opensecrets.org/lobby/clientsum.php
?id=D000031468&year=2015.

ACS's political power comes from the 2009–2010 battle over health care reform. While we would initially suspect that this would be an issue of importance to the group, the lobbying data shows differently. In a list of bills that the ACS specifically lobbied on in 2009, the ACS only reported three lobbying contacts on the Affordable Care Act, the same number of contacts that they had on a bill "to restore the traditional day of observance for Memorial Day" and far less than the 16 lobbying contacts on the Colorectal Cancer Prevention, Early Detection, and Treatment Act of 2009. Thus, much like 1994 with health care reform and the lack of congressional connection of cancer to it, we find the same pattern in 2009 with the ACS.

While the ACS also uses its political power to donate to political parties and elected officials as discussed in the previous chapter, they have to be careful to not devote too much time, energy, money, and resources to political organizing. Because their prime mission is research, education, and service to cancer patients and their families, giving too much to the political side could engender criticisms that the ACS is too political or not spending enough on their main activities and services.

Social Elements

One of the foundations of the American Cancer Society is not only its mission to provide information and awareness to the public, but the involvement of the public at large in raising funds and bringing attention to cancer. Two topics for our attention, then, are the ACS's fundraising activities and public campaigns.

Specifically in the area of fundraising, overcoming the collective action problem can be very difficult. If you haven't been directly affected by cancer or known someone who has, it is hard to understand why you would want to give your hard-earned money to the ACS, let alone any organization. Many other interest groups attempt to overcome this hurdle by offering what are termed selective benefits or incentives; these are gifts or benefits that you get by becoming a member of an organization or by giving certain amounts. You can often find these incentives during fundraising drives on public television or radio or with other interest groups like the Wounded Warrior Project. The ACS does not use this method to motivate donations; instead, they push their fundraising through events like Relay for Life, Coaches vs. Cancer, and Making Strides Against Breast Cancer Walks.

The benefit of these local events is that they can be organized by local chapters of the ACS who can utilize community and peer pressure to encourage participation and drive fundraising. Olsen, in his treatise on the collective action problem, argued that the problem would be easier to overcome in smaller groups where such peer pressure could be utilized, something the ACS is demonstrating in real life. Local Relay for Life teams are encouraged to raise funds to support their teams, thereby emphasizing the personal aspect of donating. These events can also help the ACS get their message out through local events and immediate ties.

One of the other ways in which the ACS has sought to not only increase their stature but also their fundraising coffers has been through their public appeals. Moss argues that this has been a foundational aspect of the ACS since its beginning and particularly since the Laskers and their compatriots took over control of the organization.[12] Although these public appeals do have positive aspects in informing the public as to the signs and symptoms of cancer and publicizing efforts to cure it, Moss also argues that the ACS and other cancer organizations have cultivated a "fear" of cancer primarily to drive donations, which can then be used toward finding a cure.[13] This type of public campaign "raised the ire of the organized medical professional, the American Medical Association, which accused the Society of causing mass cancerphobia."[14]

Fear is certainly a part of any public appeal of the charitable type. The fact that cancer could strike any one of us at any time or our family members is a real fear that the ACS hopes will drive donations to the organization. The criticism that Moss lays at the door of the ACS is of the use of fear to drive donations to better their organization and not necessarily find a cure. This is a criticism that is seconded by another critic, Samuel Epstein, and will be discussed further. In any case, looking at the materials that the ACS publishes today on the Internet and elsewhere, there is little of the fear mongering that Moss accuses the ACS of. Instead, the headline on the homepage of the ACS, cancer.org, is "Help Save Lives with $19 a Month"; instead of driving donations with fear, the message is rather one of hope, of saving lives. Other messages throughout their Web site also focus on more positive messages, particularly about what the ACS has done to help cancer sufferers and researchers. Today's ACS appears to be pushing a message of hope and progress rather than fear and loathing.

Scientific Elements

Despite the domination of the ACS by laypeople since the Lasker takeover, the ACS still has a strong hand in influencing the science of cancer. In fact, many of the ways in which we have previously talked about the National Cancer Institute being able to influence cancer science can also be applied to the ACS. In 2015 alone, the ACS devoted more than $150 million to cancer research; while this number is certainly smaller than the dollars the NCI has at its disposal, it is still a significant amount of funds that is highly sought after by cancer scientists. However, in the choice of which proposals to fund and which scientists to pass that money on to, the ACS can shape the priorities and topics of cancer research.

Epstein argues that much like the rest of the cancer establishment, the ACS has not been overly supportive of cancer prevention, instead focusing on efforts to find a cure.[15] This might be a fair criticism; though Epstein made this argument in 1998, in 2014, out of the $110 million available for cancer research through the ACS, only $6.9 million was given to prevention efforts. The bulk of the research dollars went to biology research, trying to understand the nature of cancer. Thus, if a research scientist is looking at this distribution of funds and would like to study prevention, they might instead change their research priorities to make it more likely that they will receive the research funding that they need for their own professional career and development.

The ACS has also influenced cancer science in other ways; for many years, they published a guide called *Unproven Methods of Cancer Management* which had the ability to influence the types of treatments the public and doctors found acceptable.[16] In addition to questionable therapies, the guide included doctors that the ACS identified as problematic. Although the listing of such doctors and treatments has long been discontinued, the ACS does make available an information sheet on "Complementary and Alternative Methods and Cancer," which is far more even-handed in the language it uses to describe questionable treatments. Not only does it explain what is meant by alternative treatments, but it also details why evidence might be difficult to come by in the case of some treatments, as well as the questions patients should ask their doctors when considering complementary and alternative treatments.

Although the danger of being somewhat "blacklisted" by the ACS no longer truly exists, because the ACS is trusted, the type of advice that is provided by the organization can shape the ways in which medical decisions are made by patients and their doctors. As a mainstream organization, alternative therapies or those pursuing such treatments will be harder to promote, particularly if there is a lack of information or research concerning them. In that sense, the ACS is a conservative organization in the type of information it will provide to the public; if the ACS all of a sudden promotes questionable practices and they turn out to be ineffective or even dangerous, the ACS risks losing its credibility.

This perspective also comes into play with the recommendations that the ACS often makes when it comes to treatment and screenings, like those for mammograms. Although the ACS has changed its guidelines over the years, it currently recommends annual mammograms beginning at age 45, whereas the U.S. Preventative Task Force says that women don't need to begin annual mammograms until 50. Epstein argues that the ACS has close ties with the mammography industry; by encouraging women to begin mammograms earlier, the mammography industry is financially benefitted. Aside from the economic implications of this argument discussed momentarily, the fact that the ACS makes recommendations of this kind can influence the direction of patient conversations and scientific research.

Economic Elements

Like Moss, Samuel Epstein has also been a strong critic of the cancer industry and especially the American Cancer Society. Epstein alleges that in addition to the close economic ties that the ACS has to the mammography industry, there are economic conflicts of interest between the ACS and the pesticide and pharmaceutical industries. Like many of the criticisms leveled by Epstein and Moss at the NCI and the ACS in the 1990s, these economic ties are hard to find today. While doctors make up far more of the board today than they did in the day of the Laskers, there are no current board members with overt ties to pharmaceuticals, mammography or radiology firms, or pesticides. Instead, the nonmedical professionals on the board represent lawyers and executives from financial service businesses. Two board members represent more well-known corporations, including Macy's and Delta Airlines.

In addition to the charge of conflict of interest, Epstein alleges that the ACS is the "world's wealthiest 'nonprofit.'"[17] He bases this allegation on data from the 1980s and 1990s which shows the ACS with hundreds of millions in reserve funds and a large real estate portfolio. Unfortunately, there is still some basis for this concern; the independent organization Charity Navigator, which monitors and rates charities based on an organization's financial health, accountability and transparency, and results, gives the ACS a score of 71.86 out of 100 based on its financial reports. Based on its 2014 financial report, the ACS spent only 59.9 percent of its funds on its services, with over a third going to fundraising expenses.[18] Compared to other similar organizations, the ACS has a poor score indeed; the Kidney Cancer Association, for example, has a score of 92.92 and the Leukemia and Lymphoma Society has a score of 76.62.[19]

The main point of the criticism leveled at the ACS by both Epstein and Moss is that because of all of these things—the lack of emphasis on prevention, the conflicts of interest, the generation of fear—the ACS is out for itself and not necessarily for a cure for cancer. In making people fear cancer and then donate in search of a cure, the ACS financially enriches itself and its board members. In 2014, the ACS's CEO made just under $1 million dollars, which does tend to justify the criticism.

As the largest and most influential cancer interest group in America, the American Cancer Society has a historical legacy of significantly affecting cancer policy and treatment. Its biggest impact has been in social and scientific terms; its push for public awareness and provision of information has the ability to portray cancer and cancer treatment in a particularly conservative light. Its approach to research has an impact on the types of projects that oncologists and researchers carry out, despite its lower level of funding. However, the ACS must proceed with caution when it expends its resources on activities other than research and patient support. Though it may like to do otherwise, the ACS must be a careful steward of its funding to preserve its organizational reputation for both the public and government officials.

The American Medical Association

The American Medical Association (AMA), like the American Cancer Society, is an interest group but an interest group of a whole different kind. Whereas the ACS can and does represent all citizens, even if they do not join the ACS or donate to it, the AMA specifically represents one group of people: doctors and those in the medical profession. It is a professional association rather than a true public interest group. Like the Congress, then, to understand why the AMA does the things it does, we must understand who they represent and the interests of those people.

The American Medical Association was formed in 1847 in order to pursue the goals of "Scientific advancement, standards for medical education, [the] launching [of] a program of medical ethics, and improved public health."[20] To understand the implications of such a program, we must remember that at that period in time, there were no standards of who could call themselves a doctor and what type of education any doctor should receive. The AMA was founded, then, to not only establish the standards of a "proper" medical education, but also to protect the doctors who had been appropriately trained and educated from the quacks and laypeople who were doctors in name only. This is essential to understanding the motivations of the AMA; they were formed to not only promote the profession but *protect* it as well. This has historically explained at least their political motivations—when policies or approaches are proposed that threaten doctors and what they do, the AMA pushes back.

Why choose to focus on the AMA if they represent doctors as a whole and not specifically oncologists? There most certainly are professional associations of oncologists and oncologic surgeons that could be focused on instead. There are two main reasons to focus on the AMA and not one of these smaller groups. First, the AMA is the largest and most powerful professional association of doctors in the United States; its political, social, scientific, and economic power far eclipses that of other specialized associations. Second, not only oncologists treat cancer. Primary care physicians are the first line of monitoring, screening, testing, diagnosing, and even treating many cancers. Before many patients see a specialist, they see a primary care or family medicine doctor; therefore, it is not just the specialty associations that are interested in cancer issues but the AMA as well.

Political Elements

The ways in which the AMA has involved itself—successfully—in health issues is indicative of the type of political power that they wield. They have been an impressively powerful organization that has played a significant role in the consideration of health care reform at all levels. For example, following the publication by a government Committee on the Costs of Medical Care in 1927 of recommendations to develop "comprehensive community medical centers" that provided care through insurance, taxation, or fee for service, the AMA came out strongly against the conclusions.[21] Believing that such a move would represent a socialism of medicine that would disrupt the contemporary doctor–patient relationship, the AMA continued to oppose New Deal plans that would provide government-sponsored health care. This all came to a head in 1939, when, following the release of "a plan for the nation's first comprehensive health program, the Justice Department began an antitrust investigation implicating the AMA, several affiliated societies and twenty-one individual physicians and hospitals from engaging in group prepayment."[22]

Although Roosevelt's 1939 plan would ultimately fail, this did not prevent the AMA from working even at the local level to stop major health care reforms. As the Kaiser Permanente system was being developed in the 1940s in California, it comprised a series of prepayment plans that drew the ire of the AMA, who accused Henry Kaiser of "unethical corporate interference in medical practice."[23] The AMA has continued its legacy of political involvement; its opposition to the Clinton health care plan in 1994 helped contribute to its ultimate demise, whereas its support in 2009 helped pave the way for the passage of the Affordable Care Act.

Like the ACS, one way to gauge their current political involvement is to look at the lobbying patterns of the AMA. Between 1998 and 2015, the AMA has spent anywhere between $9.5 million and $22.5 million on lobbying alone. In 2015, they employed or contracted 47 different lobbyists whose sole job is to pursue the interests of the AMA on Capitol Hill. These numbers are far higher than those of the ACS, demonstrating the political prowess of the group. The types of issues that the AMA lobbies on are somewhat similar to those of the ACS but strikingly different as well. While they have been interested in the Affordable Care Act and its implementation, their major issues, particularly in the past few years, surround Medicare and Medicaid and tort reform. Doctors have been profoundly interested in the Medicare and Medicaid system because the government, through the Center for Medicare and Medicaid Services (CMS), sets the reimbursement rates for services provided. Tort reform has also become an important issue for the AMA because of issues surrounding malpractice lawsuits and potential limits to what can be asked for in court.

What do these trends have to do with cancer? How much doctors are paid for treating patients on Medicare or Medicaid can greatly influence how those patients are treated and with what drugs. A 1992 Government Accountability Office (GAO) study discussed in the previous chapter found that doctors changed the way they treated cancer patients in order to maximize their Medicare/Medicaid reimbursements. How health care policies are developed and implemented does affect the treatment patients receive and the burden of costs that they are responsible for. As will be discussed in greater detail later, those with cancer have a far higher chance of declaring bankruptcy because of the high costs of cancer care, even when insurance is utilized. The fact that the AMA opposed health care reform for such a long time has inevitably affected the financial and health statuses of millions of patients, let alone those suffering from cancer.

The point to all of this is that the types of policies and programs that the AMA advocates for or against affect all of us, cancer patients included. Their political power is immense, and that makes them a force to be reckoned with, both in medicine and in politics.

Social Elements

The political status of the AMA is matched by its social standing. Its professional reputation is based on the idea that people implicitly trust their doctors and their advice. Because of this social standing, the AMA is able to make recommendations that are accepted by the medical profession and the public at large. Because of this, they are much like the ACS in that they must protect their image and reputation; one wrong move and the public's view of the entire medical profession is at stake. To that end, the types of recommendations they make and the positions they take tend to be conservative.

Despite the recommendations and initiatives that the AMA often makes, public awareness of the AMA has declined over the past decade if Google Trends is to be believed. From a high score of searches in April 2004 of 100, search frequency in the first half of 2016 has ranged between 9 and 7. More significantly, however, is where the bulk of searches for the AMA are coming from; according to Google Trends, most of the searches come from Washington, D.C. What this demonstrates is more than public awareness: the AMA has political power that perhaps eclipses its social power.

So what diminishes the social impact of the AMA? It goes back to who the AMA represents: doctors. On the other hand, the ACS represents the public at large. The AMA has never claimed to represent the general public welfare, so although it can and does publish health recommendations, at the heart of the organization is a drive to preserve professional power and legitimacy. Socially, it does what it can to enhance its reputation and therefore remains conservative as to the public actions it takes.

Scientific Elements

Once again, the matter of who is being represented comes into play as we consider the AMA's impact on the science of cancer. Doctors are in the business of treatment and curing; as such the AMA is likely to promote treatment and research into treatment rather than prevention. To that end, however, they do not sponsor or fund research like the ACS or the NCI does, instead their impact on the science of cancer is far more subtle than merely choosing which research programs to promote and fund.

One of the most prominent activities that the AMA undertakes is the publication of its flagship journals, the *Journal of the American Medical Association* (*JAMA*) and its sister publications, including the journal *JAMA Oncology*. Publication in *JAMA* is a significant event; it often represents years of hard work, dedication, research, and study. As a result of such a milestone, the authors of these works are often rewarded with increased professional prestige and standing. Such studies can often result in more grant money directed the researcher's way or academic promotion. *JAMA*, however, does not publish just any research; the studies they publish are highly respected and subjected to heavy scrutiny in the peer-review process. Although their findings are often significant or substantial, *JAMA* is not likely to publish findings that are out of the mainstream or run afoul of current thinking. *JAMA*, along with the AMA, represent the mainstream of medical knowledge and opinion; one does not get published in *JAMA* by going against the flow.

Through the mechanism of research publication, the AMA can have a significant impact on what science is published and ultimately given medical sanction. This is just the case that was encountered in the cases of Laetrile and vitamin C discussed earlier in this book. This obviously has pros and cons; it is good in that the science that is published is quite concrete and well founded. To provide suspicious or unfounded medical advice would come close to medical malpractice. However, there is often good research that either goes unpublished or published in lower-tier journals because of this conservative bent. It is in this way that the AMA, through *JAMA* and *JAMA Oncology*, can shape the knowledge of the medical profession.

One additional way in which the AMA shapes scientific behavior is through its codification of medical ethics. As one of the founding missions of the AMA, these guidelines provide the very concrete rules by which doctors practice and perform their work. No doctor would wish to run afoul of the AMA ethical guidelines for fear of being blacklisted or accumulating a poor professional reputation.

Economic Elements

The American Medical Association is very much an economic organization—they are interested in protecting doctors and their livelihoods. This should not be construed to be a positive or negative statement, merely a statement of fact. The fact is that there are hundreds of professional organizations across the United States that represent almost every profession or career that there is. These organizations are formed to look after the interests of their members; this is only natural. The AMA derives its economic power partially from the social status of doctors and the medical profession, as well as the economic impact that such a profession has.

Many of the policy positions that the AMA has taken that were detailed earlier have a clear economic implication for doctors. If health care reform that instituted a single payer system or something approximating it had ever been implemented, the government would have assumed a large chunk of control of the amount of money that doctors could charge for their services and thus their income. Medicaid and Medicare reimbursements similarly affect the bottom line. This economic power is clearly tied and parlayed into political power; most of the large-scale policies that will affect the medical profession are those that are controlled by, if not the federal government, then by state and local governments. The economic power of the AMA is only reinforced by the incredible amount that they spend on lobbying efforts year in and year out. Like the ACS, the AMA cannot be seen to spend too much on governmental affairs, so the fact that they can spend somewhere around $20 million a year on lobbying is indicative of the resources they have at their disposal.

The American Medical Association is a politically and economically powerful organization. They do an excellent job of representing their members, just as we would expect of any organization that is created to do so. With respect to their influence on issues relating to cancer, they have the ability to shape (or help shape) the way and how much doctors are paid for their services; if a chemotherapeutic drug could be administered in the doctor's office but the reimbursement rate is lower than at the hospital, a doctor might needlessly send the patient to a hospital. The AMA can shape mainstream medical and public opinion about appropriate treatments, screenings, and diagnoses through its well-known and well-respected publications. The social and economic standing of doctors props up the political power, reinforcing the status of the AMA in Washington as a force to be reckoned with and respected.

The Pharmaceutical Industry

In 2015, a young pharmaceutical CEO, Martin Shkreli, made headline news when his company, Turing Pharmaceuticals, raised the price of a treatment for toxoplasmosis by more than 5500 percent from $13.50 a pill to $750 a pill.[24] What made Shkreli's case even more infuriating for much of the public and even the political system was his apparent aloofness when appearing at a congressional hearing called to investigate the sudden increase in the drug's cost. While Shkreli is currently facing charges of fraud, unfortunately, the case of Daraprim, the toxoplasmosis drug, is not the only one of its kind; the pharmaceutical industry has faced increasing criticism for its pricing methodology that has treatments for some diseases costing upwards of $100,000 a year.

Cancer drugs have come under particular scrutiny, especially as it has come to light that being diagnosed with cancer greatly increases one's chances of having to declare bankruptcy. Ubel et al. detail just a few examples of these increasing costs: a Medicare patient facing colorectal cancer may pay up to $8,800 in out-of-pocket costs for a 10-month course of treatment with bevacizumab.[25] In Massachusetts, out-of-pocket costs for a patient with breast cancer could be as high as $55,250 with a high-deductible insurance plan. The price of many of these oncology drugs have risen 5- to 10-fold since 2000 alone.[26] Even for those patients with insurance plans, out-of-pocket costs for deductibles and travel to and from oncologists can spell financial disaster that only death will be able to erase.

The reasons why the cost of cancer drugs has risen faster than inflation are many and complicated. Howard et al. lay out several reasons, including reference pricing and required drug discounts and price supports.[27] Reference pricing is the practice of looking at the drugs that are already on the market and setting the price of new drugs 10 to 20 percent higher, even if the benefits they offer are no more than the benefits of the drugs already available. Utilizing this method allows pharmaceutical manufacturers to claim that the price of the drug is within the range of currently available treatments. Further, drug companies are required to provide discounts to low-income patients so the cost of such provision must be taken into account when setting the sale price as a whole. Siddiqui and Rajkumar identify other reasons for the high costs, including the costs of three phases of trials and then regulatory approval, something Kantarjian et al., as well as the pharmaceutical industry, would agree with.[28] PhRMA, the Pharmaceutical Research and Manufacturers of America, the industry interest group, states that that average cost for bringing one drug to market is $2.6 billion; if the costs of drugs are decreased, there is the potential of stifling innovation and research and development, which would ultimately harm patients in the end.[29]

Effective drugs produced by the pharmaceutical industry are an integral part of cancer treatment. In addition to surgery and radiotherapy, chemotherapy is an important part of treating most types of cancer. The influence of the pharmaceutical industry not only in setting drug prices but in creating drugs to begin with is quite significant. Without the research and development breakthroughs that these companies continually invest in and shepherd from trial to trial to the FDA, many of the advanced treatments we now have for cancer would not exist. Just as important as doctors are in the treatment of cancer, drugs, the tools for which doctors reach for, are equally important.

Political Elements

For an industry that has such scientific and economic significance, it's not surprising that much of that influence is translated into the political arena. Not only is the pharmaceutical industry interested in the rules and regulations for drug approval or the laws (or lack thereof) controlling prices, they are also interested in Washington, D.C., for one very big reason: Medicare. Medicare, government health insurance for the elderly, is the biggest payer for anticancer drugs in the United States, with Medicaid falling at number three.[30] And with the baby boomer generation set to retire at record numbers in the coming years, Medicare represents a significant portion not only of the health care industry, but also an important source of income for drug companies. Because of this, there are two major areas of policy that the industry is deeply involved in: the ability of Medicare to negotiate lower drug prices and the ability of patients to acquire drugs from overseas.

Current law does not allow Medicare to negotiate bulk prices of drugs on behalf of its beneficiaries. As we've discussed previously, in the developed world, this is an odd situation; the ability of a government to negotiate on behalf of a large part of the population does tend to drive down overall prices, particularly with the threat that the government will not cover the prices of those drugs at all. Kantarjian et al. estimate that by simply allowing Medicare to negotiate with drug companies would save the United States $40 to $80 billion a year.[31] To date, policy makers have been unwilling to take such a drastic move, particularly with the lobbying power that PhRMA as an interest group and the drug companies individually wield (to be discussed later). However, these companies must also be careful not to play politics and raise drug prices so high so as to force the hand of the federal government.

The second major policy element that pharma is interested in is the inability of patients to acquire drugs from abroad at significantly cheaper prices. Stories about the pursuit of prescription drugs from across the border abound in movies like *Dallas Buyers Club* which focuses on HIV/AIDS medications. Although drug companies ostensibly claim that they oppose the move due to concerns over patient safety, the Canadian government's Patented Medicine Prices Review Board found in 2011 that patients in America pay 100 percent more for patented drugs than elsewhere.[32] PhRMA phrases their opposition as follows:

> In the 1980s, when the US drug supply was open to foreign medicines, many women taking birth control were getting pregnant. After many complaints and investigations, it was discovered they were taking counterfeit pills of foreign origin. Members of Congress took action to help prevent this from happening again and passed a bill called the Prescription Drug Marketing Act. This bill closed the US drug supply system to help prevent foreign counterfeit drugs from getting in the hands of American patients who rely on safe medicines to live longer, healthier, and more productive lives.[33]

What's more important than the policy battles that pharmaceutical companies have an interest in is what type of power they possess and wield that allows them to get their way in these debates. Much like the AMA, the economic power of the pharmaceutical industry has direct impact on the political power that the industry can wield through lobbying. If we focus just on PhRMA, the industry interest group, and not the individual drug companies themselves, we get an idea of the type of attention the industry devotes to politics. Peaking in 2009 with the consideration of the Affordable Care Act, PhRMA spent $26.1 million on lobbying alone. That number has fallen to $18.9 million in 2015, but even given that, they still have 137 registered lobbyists in Washington, D.C.[34]

PhRMA has also made its presence known in donating to political candidates. For the 2016 election cycle, through July 2016, PhRMA had contributed $765,000 to various candidates and political groups. Although they gave $2,735 to the Democratic National Committee, the vast majority of these contributions were to arms of the Republic National Committee or Republican-affiliated groups.[35] This continues a pattern established in the 2014 election cycle of overwhelming dedication of funds toward Republicans, including $7,500 to the Republican Party of Kentucky, where Senate Majority Leader Mitch McConnell was facing a staunch Democratic challenger.

These numbers represent only the lobbying and donation activities of PhRMA; between 2015 and 2016, the health industry in general ranks sixth in the amount of money it has spent on lobbying and political donations. In the top 20 of contributors within the health sector are six different pharmaceutical companies (Exoxemis, Pfizer, Amgen, Celgene, Eli Lilly, and Sanofi). These figures demonstrate the power of the pharmaceutical industry within politics and why they continually find success in supporting or blocking particular policy measures. Particularly because there is no government ability to negotiate for lower drug prices, most of the drug companies can count on higher profit margins within the United States, and they therefore seek to protect their economic prospects via political means.

Social Elements

We started this section by detailing the case of Martin Shkreli and the exorbitant price increase his company made on a single drug. Cases like these stimulate popular backlash when the media publicizes these salacious stories. However, despite the steep increase in drugs in recent years, the public still seems more than willing to pay these costs, even if the most you can expect from them is a few months of added life expectancy. For instance, when a proposal for Oregon's Medicaid program intended to limit the coverage of cancer drugs, public outcry meant that the proposal was ultimately dead on arrival.[36] Despite our moral and political outrage at the ways in which the pharmaceutical industry is supposedly gouging us, patients are still willing to pay whatever price in order to live.

Part of the reason that pharmaceutical companies can get away with setting higher drug prices is because of the mechanisms available to patients to reduce the cost that they ultimately pay. For many people, this comes in the form of health insurance, which, after the passage of the Affordable Care Act, must cover all costs once an out-of-pocket maximum is reached. This means that many Americans don't realize just how much that pill they are popping or drug that is dripping into their veins actually costs. Further, companies offer deep discounts required by law to low-income patients, which some argue is part of the problem of high costs in the first place. These types of discounts include assistance provided by the drug companies directly. These price supports not only lower the ultimate costs for patients and inoculate them somewhat from experiencing ultra-high prices, but also can engender goodwill among the public that can serve to blunt any criticism that arises.

One effect of these high prices does have the potential for stoking a social outrage against high drug prices and the drug companies: cancer patients are at a higher risk of bankruptcy.[37] This is a very real effect of high costs, and as the number of Americans who are diagnosed with cancer increases, it is something that will affect more and more people, even those who do have health insurance. Aside from the drug costs, copayments for specialist doctors' visits and travel to and from oncologists, particularly if people are located in rural parts of the country, adds up quickly. And unfortunately, this financial insolvency can contribute to a higher risk of death in these same cancer patients.[38]

Unfortunately, social outrage brought on by these isolated publicized cases of high drug prices is only temporary. When the media highlights these exceptional cases, public interest and pressure do rise, but that increased attention is not sustained. Without a high amount of social pressure exerted over a significant period, drug companies know that if they can weather the momentary storm of criticism, they can go on charging the rates they want for drugs, particularly with the political insulation that their lobbying and donation dollars ensure. Added to this is the public willingness to pay and the fact that doctors continue to prescribe; because the choice is often either pay for the drug or face death (or at least a quicker death), patients make the choice to pay. The drug companies get their money and there is no incentive to change their pricing behavior. Add in the fact that doctors are often encouraged to prescribe the latest and greatest in available treatments, regardless of cost, and patients are willing to go into debt. Unfortunately, the choice of whether to pay or not is not much of a choice at all.

Scientific Elements

At the end of the day, science drives the development of new and revolutionary drugs. Without understanding the chemical, biological, or genetic components of cancer, nobody would know what to even target with potential compounds. Discoveries of genes specifically tied to cancer, like the BRCA1 and BRCA2 genes, initiate the search for drugs that can target those genes directly. The increasing ability of oncologists to genetically type and differentiate different cancers has led to a whole new set of medications. In this way, the development of new drugs and the activity of the pharmaceutical industry are intimately tied to the science of the day.

There is an interesting relationship between a market and innovation, however. Moss details a long history of how various dominating businesses have discouraged the development of new and revolutionary products like the VCR or even digital recording technologies.[39] The thought is that the introduction of new technologies will drive current companies to either adapt and change or perish; for many companies incapable of changing and keeping up with the times, their ultimate fate is to simply die. We can see this with any number of tech companies, from AOL to Hewlett Packard. Betting on one technology or not moving quick enough to capture a new market portends their ultimate doom.

A similar line of thought is at work in pharmaceuticals, according to Moss. The development of new and revolutionary drugs is likely not only to cost billions of dollars in research and development, but could hurt other facets of their business. Thus, Moss argues, big pharma companies are likely to, and probably have already, stifled true innovation that could change the very nature of cancer care. Although it is hard to find evidence supporting such an accusation, the line of inquiry is easily understood. In fact, the development of entirely new molecular entities (a class of new drug) has fallen, with the FDA approving fewer and fewer. Instead, many of the new drugs approved by the FDA for use in the United States are drugs that slightly improve or build upon previous treatments, leading to marginal benefits over previously available drugs. In fact, Howard et al. find that though there is a correlation between higher costs of cancer drugs and overall survival time (the higher the cost, the longer the survival time), their research finds that newer drugs *do not* provide greater survival benefits than older drugs.[40]

The phenomenon of higher drug prices has not gone unnoticed by oncologists. Ubel and colleagues have argued that doctors should talk to their patients about the costs of drugs as if they were a true side effect like vomiting, nausea, or diarrhea.[41] Other oncologists have suggested ways in which the cost issue could be dealt with, including the ability of the federal government to negotiate lower prices for Medicare. One set of oncologists argue that one way to reduce costs for cancer drugs would be to base the costs on the added life expectancy that those drugs will give a patient.[42] Although this would be one way to stimulate research into revolutionary new drugs that could give doctors and patients a leg up over older treatments, the measurement of life expectancy through clinical trials puts the science of drug trials at a premium. As we have discussed previously, not all clinical trials are alike; most have methodologies that are wide ranging and difficult to compare from one study to another. If drug trials are suddenly used to determine drug costs, what sort of methodology should be mandated? Would there need to be a placebo group, even if that means one group of patients suffering from cancer will receive *no* treatment whatsoever? What are the ethics involved with such a practice? Using science to discover new drugs is one thing; using it to set prices leads us into an ethical and moral wonderland with no rabbit hole to escape out of.

Economic Elements

"The purpose of research from the point of view of business is, and always has been, to facilitate profit making."[43] At the end of the day, making drugs and selling them, although we would like to think it's about saving lives, is actually about making money. Businesses and corporations exist for the sole purpose of turning a profit for their investors. While there are certainly nonprofit labs across the world that are putting good work into developing new drugs, the vast majority of drugs that come onto the market, including cancer drugs, are produced by large drug manufacturers.

This is not to say that this is a bad situation to have; to quote Gordon Gekko, "Greed is good." If a company could not make a profit off a product, there would be little incentive to innovate and meet market demand. For better or for worse, the market conditions of capitalism, of supply and demand, of the invisible hand, have largely worked. Further, if drug companies can make profits off of currently available drugs, that means even more money is available for new research and a continuing pipeline of innovation.

Whatever your political or economic position is on the role of pharmaceutical businesses specifically and big business in general, we must acknowledge that the fact that pharma is out to make money is a guiding principle affecting not only the selling of drugs but the development as well. Some people have criticized the lack of research into treatments for cancers or diseases that less frequently afflict the population; instead, companies focus their research on those diseases that will likely allow them to sell a high volume of drugs rather than a small number for a rare disease. This is one purpose of government funding for research and development; where there is no business incentive to develop but there is a need, a market failure occurs and the government steps in. This drive for profit is another way in which innovation can be stifled, as pharmaceutical-backed researchers aim to develop drugs and treatments that are incremental and all but guaranteed to turn a profit rather than focus on new, untried, and untested treatments that will probably go nowhere.[44]

Economic incentives are a double-edged sword. Companies are encouraged to develop products for which there is a market and to continually improve those drugs so they can sell more at higher prices. But in order to guarantee a profit, they are more conservative in the research and development choices they make, sometimes foreclosing promising lines of research. Further, the incredible amount of dollars that the industry brings in allows them to wield political and social power with such adeptness as to insulate themselves from major policy changes that could possibly affect their bottom line. Unfortunately, in such a situation, the poor economic conditions of those suffering from cancer matter less than a reduction in profit for one of the big drug companies.

Like the American Medical Association, the economic prowess of the pharmaceutical industry feeds their ability to pursue political goals. This can all be tempered, however, by the social outrage that can be stirred up when the costs of drugs rise astronomically or people continue to have to declare bankruptcy in order to treat their cancer. Thus, pharmaceutical companies must pay special attention to social elements of their business, taking care to avoid bad publicity and make drugs available at lower costs to certain populations.

Conclusions

In reviewing the actors discussed in this chapter, one could get the impression that the actions of the ACS, the AMA, and the pharmaceutical industry are somewhat muddled, or to use a less technical term, "icky." They pursue their very real material benefits, even if that means other groups are likely to suffer. They use their social and economic standing to protect certain groups over others. Their actions can sometimes directly harm (or at least not benefit), the sickest and most vulnerable among us. But at the end of the day, that could be said about any actor in this book. What all of these groups are doing are acting out of the best interest of the people whom they represent. Isn't that what all of us want, really? To have someone to represent us and to be our voice?

Another way to look at this issue is through the lens of Dr. Jekyll and Mr. Hyde. In one sense, all of these actors benefit us in some ways; the ACS raises funds and distributes them for cancer research, doctors are the experts we turn to when our lives are in danger, and the drug companies provide the doctors the treatments that can save our lives. Those are all really good things that we are lucky to have in society. On the other hand, they can use their influence and economic, social, and political power to benefit themselves at the expense of others, including patients. At the end of the day, they are not all truly good nor truly bad, but who among us ever is?

This chapter demonstrates the intertwining of political, social, scientific, and economic power. The American Cancer Society uses its social standing to make the voice of cancer patients and their families heard. Doctors use their social and economic standing combined with scientific expertise to protect their professional reputation. And drug companies use their scientific knowledge to produce economic benefits that allow them entry into the political process. These dimensions rarely stand on their own but are used to bolster one another for the cancer industry. Cancer is not solely a medical or scientific problem, it is a political one and for many patients, truly an economic one.

CHAPTER SEVEN

Lessons

As I begin writing this chapter, I find myself in the midst of training for an event much like the ones discussed in the previous chapter that the American Cancer Society puts on. It's an annual half-marathon run called Spirit of Survival that raises funds for the local cancer center and has a heavy emphasis on awareness of cancer issues. As a runner for over a decade now, this certainly isn't the first or the last run of this sort that I'll train for. In the past, I've run nearly a dozen half-marathons, many of them at Walt Disney World, the proceeds of which have traditionally gone to the Leukemia and Lymphoma Society. I never really connected my running with cancer when I first started; for me, it represents a challenge to myself, racing not against other people but my own brain and my own previous times. Out on the course, you'll see dozens of people in their purple Team in Training shirts who are specifically running to raise funds for the Leukemia and Lymphoma Society and even at Spirit of Survival, people will wear signs dedicating their runs to people with cancer or who have had cancer. In fact, it really wasn't until quite recently that I connected what I do for fun and fitness with the cancer movement at all.

While big events like marathons or half-marathons raise comparatively small amounts of money for cancer programs and research, the fact that so many people are now participating in them does send some very important messages. Yes, people are more concerned about their health and fitness level than ever before, and running is one way to manage that. But why has it become so important? In addition to rising levels of obesity in America, studies have consistently shown that being in shape does help decrease people's chances of getting cancer. In fact, most people who go to these types of events are not professional athletes who spend their careers training and running, they are normal everyday people just looking to get in shape. Additionally, in simply seeing the number of runners who are dedicating their runs to someone with cancer, you get a feel for just how deeply cancer affects a community. That people will spend their Saturday mornings getting up at the crack of dawn to go train for a race simply because other people cannot is a testament to the hurt but also the hope that cancer and cancer research bring. To be able to support a community by the mere act of running, instead of fighting against cancer, is a powerful motivator to run.

For me, however, a race that used to be a challenge, a personal motivator of sorts, has become a monument of sorts in my head. Not only will the Spirit of Survival be my first half-marathon in three years due to a slew of injuries, but coming as it is on the tail end of preparing this book, it is a monument to the people deeply involved in the war (or the moonshot) against cancer. The millions of patients, families, doctors, researchers, and yes, politicians, who have sought for so long against such great odds to fight such a deadly disease. The war will probably not be won tomorrow, but so long as people keep fighting, and running, we are well on our way.

This book has detailed numerous hurdles that keep the government from creating a comprehensive, cohesive, and effective policy against cancer. The pressures of government and representation represent crosswinds, pulling policy makers and elected officials in different directions. This chapter will serve not only to summarize the findings of this research but to draw lessons for those so intimately involved in the fight against cancer, the patients, the doctors, and the politicians. Although we cannot change the institutions of government to make policy making for cancer, or any other public problem, easier, in recognizing our shortcomings, perhaps we can point the direction for future efforts in solving the problem.

Where We Are

We've come a long way in our knowledge about cancer since the beginning of the 20th century and even since the war on cancer was declared in 1971. While we still don't know everything about carcinogenesis or what makes a normal cell turn against its biology, we have begun to identify particular genes that make cells go haywire and begun to create defenses against them. We've recognized the dangers in many environmental exposures, including asbestos, tobacco, and even the sun and tanning beds. But the science of what contributes or not to one's chance of getting cancer is ever more muddled. Will sitting behind a desk lead to cancer sometime down the road? How many miles do I need to run a day to reduce my chances of cancer? How many fruits and vegetables per day does someone need? What's the value of wine, coffee, or alcohol in preventing or contributing to cancer? These questions represent the significant amount of uncertainty that still remains in our knowledge about cancer.

As we've discovered, scientific uncertainty is a necessary by-product of the scientific process. The ways in which science is conducted today greatly shape scientific knowledge and research agendas; academic scientists seeking publications or grant money in order to be promoted and receive greater recognition for their work rarely pursue questionable avenues of research. The types of grant money available direct researchers to study areas that are of interest to the providers; for example, Chapters 1 and 2 demonstrate that although the Department of Defense (DOD) has been a significant distributor of research funds, those receiving the dollars must conform their research to the motivations of the DOD. The debate among the cancer community of whether the focus should be on prevention or treatment of cancer also affects these lines of research; most of the organizations we've discussed here, including the National Cancer Institute and the American Cancer Society, provide significantly more funds for research into treatment so scientists examining prevention are often shortchanged.

All of these crosscurrents have contributed to the strained relationship between science and government. Government agencies have their own priorities for cancer policy that scientists needing funds try to match, but the science often points in directions other than where the government wants to go. The uncertainty and mixed findings that are hallmarks of the scientific process makes communicating between policy makers and scientists difficult; policy makers do not understand why they can't get concrete findings and data, and the scientists don't understand why policy makers don't listen to their advice. Too often, this leads to contentious debates and difficulty in identifying best practices and the best policy to implement.

The burden of most of these debates is usually placed within bureaucracies whose job it is to interpret law and implement a policy in the best way possible. The bureaucracies we have discussed, primarily in Chapter 2, are the unsung players in cancer policy. Although most people would not recognize the name if they heard it, the National Cancer Institute is a vital player in cancer research and treatment, providing the largest amount of funds for research available. This money is vital to the doctors, researchers, and academics who have devoted their careers to understanding and preventing cancer. Thus, while the public may not be aware of what they do, they have had a huge impact on the science and understanding of cancer. The Environmental Protection Agency, similarly, has left its mark in the types and amounts of potentially cancer-causing chemicals that Americans are exposed to on a routine basis. It is their responsibility to ensure the health of the public, but all too often, their mission is highly political with science used as fodder for debate rather than decisions. Because the regulations on which their job is premised are so important to the bottom line of business and industry, the EPA is caught between their duty to protect the environment and public health and the need to satisfy powerful political overlords and economic interests. This was clearly indicated in the analysis of regulations in Chapter 3, which showed that patterns of regulations are quite susceptible to political currents, particularly the split between the Republican and Democratic parties.

The Food and Drug Administration also has a fascinating role to play. Like the EPA, they ensure that carcinogenic compounds are not exposed to the American public through the foods they eat, but they also have the final say in the drugs that are available to treat diseases like cancer. Through their stepped-up efforts in the second half of the 20th century to require data on safety and effectiveness, the FDA singlehandedly established the science and practice of drug trials. Although this has often contributed to disputes between the FDA and the NCI as to the testing of cancer drugs and standards for effectiveness, the FDA has allowed for certain amounts of flexibility and public input into the decisions that they have made. However, because the standards of approval and testing have become so rigorous, it is generally only large pharmaceutical companies that can get a product from research and development to testing and approval; thus the FDA is sensitive to industry concerns, making the politics of the agency somewhat subtle but still apparent.

We often expect that politics might affect major players the most, especially the president. Day in and day out, presidents are placed at the center of American politics, sometimes driving the discussion and sometimes merely reacting to it. But no matter which way the political winds are blowing, the public still thinks of the president as the most powerful politician and policy maker in America. That could certainly be debated, but what is surprising about the findings presented here is that the amount of politics and political calculations involved when presidents discuss cancer is surprisingly low; this is not to say that politics is completely absent, but compared to other actors, the politics of cancer is minimal when it comes to the president. Instead, cancer has become a social issue in two ways. First, presidents have historically responded to increased societal pressure to act on cancer. Both Lyndon B. Johnson and Richard Nixon are prime examples of this phenomenon—for them the pressure came from Mary Lasker and the American Cancer Society. Second, presidents have also pursued cancer policy when they have been personally affected by the disease. Whether it's been to humanize the president or enhance a personal connection with the American public, presidents have been apt to invoke their own stories and experiences with cancer in their families, conditioning their chances of reacting to cancer issues.

Where the politics of cancer were somewhat reduced within the presidency, when Congress has considered issues related to cancer, their actions have been highly political. Members of Congress have sought to use cancer to their political advantage, specifically to advantage their reelection efforts. They have held hearings about local cancer clusters and examined policy issues from a local perspective. Like the president, however, members of Congress do respond to social and, particularly, media pressure. When public concern about cancer is higher or when the media focus has increased, Congress has tended to hold more hearings on cancer policy. The analysis of congressional hearings in Chapter 5 clearly shows certain periods of action that relate to public pressure (the 1960s), media pressure (1980s), and social pressure (1990s). Added to this is the wide variety of topics that members have been interested in. Members of Congress seem to get their fingers in everywhere: policy, oversight, science and medical advice, and even economics, particularly when it comes to their state or district. Of course, as we've discussed previously, these types of concerns are natural and to be expected from those individuals who we have selected to be our political eyes and ears.

The final set of actors that we have sought to examine includes the other members of the cancer community, in particular, the American Cancer Society, the American Medical Association, and the pharmaceutical industry. As for what can be said about all three of these actors is that no single influence, political, social, scientific, or economic, stands out about their actions; instead, all are intertwined, feeding one into the other. For example, the American Cancer Society's main power comes from the fact that it is a public interest group with a large amount of members and deep fundraising coffers. While they have the ability to influence the science of cancer through the funding they give to research, the social power contributes to their political power on Capitol Hill. And although the ACS is still actively involved in lobbying members of Congress and promoting cancer policy, their entre into politics has receded since the days of Mary Lasker, the dominant policy entrepreneur of her time.

For both the AMA and the pharmaceutical industry, instead of social power leading to political influence, their astounding success in the political sphere can be attributed to their economic standing. The AMA, as a leading voice of all doctors in the United States, has been a political tour de force; they have been fiercely protective of doctors' domains and very successful at it. The economic prowess of doctors and their social respect-ability lend the AMA reputation and ability to effectively organize and act as one voice in political spheres. And although the AMA is primarily influential in politics and economics, they also have the ability to influence the science of cancer in the form of their flagship publication the *Journal of the American Medical Association*. The pharmaceutical industry largely mirrors this pattern; they have the ability to drive science and research, but their real power comes from their economic dominance, which allows them to be incredibly influential and active in politics. In fact, these two ele-ments feed off of each other; pursuing policy that is favorable to drug companies like the inability of Americans to procure drugs from else-where increases the bottom line of these companies, which in turn gives them more political clout.

And what is the overall cause of the behaviors observed by all of these actors? In general, they are acting based on what is good for them or their agency. While this was something that was first encountered specifically in Chapter 5 on the Congress, the same could be said for any of the actors in this book. Bureaucrats in the NCI, the EPA, or the FDA may be acting in response to certain laws or initiatives; however, the *way* in which they respond is greatly conditioned on what they think is in their best interest. For example, as Chapter 3 demonstrated, the FDA often acts to uphold a particular reputation they have for protecting the public good; being too careless or reckless in approving drugs could very well do damage to that public reputation and cause Americans to lose faith in the agency. The EPA has reacted to changes in partisan balance in Congress and the White House, and while that might be expected based on shifts from Republicans to Democrats and vice versa, they must also protect their organizational image as being responsive to political concerns. At the end of the day, no bureaucratic agency or department in the U.S. government can act with-out sufficient resources, or in other words, money. Because every agency competes annually for their share of the U.S. budget, all agencies, includ-ing the ones discussed here, must protect their standing among politi-cians in order to protect the potential resources they may be given.

It's far easier to see the self-interested motivations of the other actors in this book; presidents want to be seen as responsive and effective to public concerns. That they react when the public is concerned is to be expected. That they use an issue like cancer, one that you can practically do no wrong on, is natural. Members of Congress protect their interests by using can-cer issues to their own advantage. The pharmaceutical industry wants larger profits and revenues so they act to maximize their returns. Doctors want to protect their industry and ability to practice, and the American Cancer Society is acting on behalf of not only cancer patients but those interested in researching, treating, and preventing cancer. Unfortunately, out of all of these institutions, the only one that could be argued to be acting specifically on behalf of those who are suffering the most is the ACS and even then, their behaviors could be questioned. The sad conclusion to be drawn, then, is that while all of these organizations and individuals might *want* to cure cancer, their cross-cutting motivations and desires often prevent them from working more fully together. Such different motivations lead all of these people to not want to work together but to work separately for the good of their own patrons and benefactors.

In thinking about all of these patterns, one way to not only roughly summarize the findings but draw conclusions about which factor—political, social, scientific, or economic—has been most important is to do a bit of "rough justice." Table 7.1 lists the different actors that have been discussed in this book along with our four analytical dimensions. Based on the findings of this research, I have rated the influence of each category—political, social, scientific, or economic—as being either low, medium, or high. On its own, Table 7.1 provides a quick summary of what this book has found. But to take it one step further, we can assign a number value to the terms low, medium, and high and then sum each column to determine how many "points" each dimension has. If low has a value of 1, medium, 2, and high a value of 3, the column totals result in 19 points for politics, 15 for social, 19 for scientific, and 17 for economic.

Based on this, it would seem that the four analytical dimensions used in this research are on fairly equal footing as far as relevance and

Table 7.1   Overall Summary and Analysis

Actor	Political	Social	Scientific	Economic
NCI	Low	Low	High	Medium
EPA	High	Low	Medium	High
FDA	Medium	Medium	High	High
President	Medium	High	Low	Low
Congress	High	High	High	High
ACS	Medium	High	High	Low
AMA	High	Low	Medium	Low
Pharma	High	Low	Medium	High
Point Totals	**19**	**15**	**19**	**17**

importance, with politics and science taking the lead. This suggests that the most important influences in determining cancer policy have been both political and scientific elements; whereas the finding that the science of cancer is important is not at all surprising, the fact that politics can claim equal status with it is. For those involved in cancer policy and research and development, the fact that the politics of cancer is often ignored can be considered a shortfall.

Based not only on the conclusions that can be drawn from Table 7.1 but also the fact that institutional behavior toward cancer policy in the United States is often driven by self-interested motivations, the next section offers some advice for policy makers, scientists, and patients based on the findings in this book.

Lessons

A certain colloquial saying goes "Don't hate the player, hate the game." This is usually used in a very different situation than this book or even in the context of cancer, but there is a lesson for patients, researchers, and policy makers in the saying. The only way to win a game, any game, is to either understand the rules and play them better than anybody else or to completely upend the rules and create new ones. Unfortunately, the institutions of Washington, the rules by which the political game is played, are not likely to change anytime soon. As such, the main lesson to be learned from this research is that cancer policy is very much a product of the political game, and in order to be successful in the arena, we must all recognize, understand, and learn to play by the rules, even if cancer has no rules to play by.

Policy Makers

Policy makers have, perhaps, the easiest job of all when it comes to changing the way they behave with regard to cancer. They not only have the power of the purse, but the ability to change the ways in which that purse is divvied up and handed out. They can change the way grants are disbursed and for what purposes. They can give more money to prevention efforts. They can take legislative steps to fix some of the problems that affect cancer policy. In short, policy makers have the ability, if not the willingness, to solve many of the conundrums facing cancer policy in the 21st century.

In examining the lessons of this book and the summary earlier, politics is clearly a driving factor, if not the biggest and most significant, in the design and construction of cancer policy. Everything from regulations to research and development has a political, even partisan, twinge to it. Although it might appear as if there is a bipartisan, nonpolitical alliance against cancer, there is no such thing when it comes to the different components of policy. The problem, then, is not an unwillingness to fight cancer but an inability to clearly see cancer policy as a conglomeration of other policy areas that must each work in concert to make a dent in the modern cancer epidemic. It's not that they don't want to end cancer, it's that they simply can't.

This is perhaps the most dangerous problem of all; if we only tackle cancer from one direction—for instance, treatment—we will never prevent people from experiencing it in the first place. If we only focus on the most frequently occurring cancers, we'll never understand and know how to treat more rare forms of it. The inability to see the pieces of the whole, the trees through the forest, means that American cancer policy will never form a coherent whole that will make elimination of cancer an actual possibility.

So why can't politicians see the details and connect the dots? There are certainly many reasons this is the case, and while this is not the place to hash out those ideas and theories, there are some hints of why this must be so. The hyperlocal focus of members of Congress pushes them to focus on smaller pieces of the pie, of what can be done at a local level instead of what should be done at a national level. The all-consuming partisan warfare that infects many parts of the policy process limits what people think the government could or should do. In fact, at the end of the day, this really is a question of what government should be able to do. If you believe that government should be limited and small in scale, then perhaps cancer is not a policy issue you believe government should be meddling in. If you believe that the role of the government should be to ensure a certain level of treatment or ability, then ensuring public health might be an area you want government involvement in. Although these are obviously disagreements in principle that cannot be easily rectified, the two-headed monster of beliefs that tears at the government makes it hard to do anything on a whole to begin with.

The extent to which partisan polarization has affected this country politically and otherwise cannot be denied. Budget politics have suffered, and the ability to create policy based on evidence and data rather than fear and divisiveness have preempted efforts to improve outcomes across the country. The mere fact that increased polarization has led to less productivity has reduced the chances of Congress moving bills into law in the first place. And while the causes of this polarization cannot be discussed in further detail here, it is obviously a significant factor in the failure of policy making all around. The founding fathers may have wanted to make it difficult for Congress to affect laws, but they didn't want to make it impossible.

There is another side to this argument, however. Even if Congress is not actively writing law and making policy, the actions of members through hearings and budgeting and the actions of the president in carrying out those laws do mean that progress is still being made. It may simply be that members of Congress see no need to pass laws about cancer, instead preferring the status quo. Indeed, Vice President Joe Biden's moonshot to end cancer does not call for any new legislation, only more funding and more stylistic changes in how cancer research and development is carried out. This has continued trends since Bill Clinton to focus more on the mechanics of cancer policy rather than the content.

If there is any lesson to be learned by policy makers, then, it is that despite the polarization, despite the partisan aspects, and despite their initial inclinations to think local, they must see the problem that is cancer from an overarching perspective that incorporates all aspects of cancer policy and not just bits here and there. Policy makers and politicians must think globally in attacking cancer and realize that significant decisions or policies in seemingly unrelated areas may have consequences, perhaps even dire consequences, from those suffering from cancer or at risk of it. It is the realization that cancer does not stop at the hospital's edge but continues into our communities, our economies, and our society that policy makers must come to understand if we are ever to overcome the other problems associated with making policy today.

Doctors, Researchers, and the Scientific Community

When training doctors, scientists, and academics, one of the toughest subjects to broach and focus on is the fact that individuals should remain as objective and neutral as possible. This is often difficult for individuals to achieve because one, we're human, and two, we may not always recognize our implicit biases. In order to avoid subjectivity, we have to be aware of the ways in which we are subjective. Doctors and scientists may already recognize some of their own biases, specifically as with regard to their specialties or research, but there has to be greater awareness of the professional culture and biases that emerge within it. This means that those engaging in cancer research should acknowledge that as a whole, it is easy for research agendas to be influenced and swayed by the dominant lines of thought of the day. Instead of letting the research findings direct future paths for research, what this book has shown is that too often, professional subjectivity puts researchers on a path to particular inquiries that are currently favored.

This also means that doctors and those researching cancer treatments should understand their own predilection to treatment instead of prevention. This particular bias has led to a systematic de-emphasis on prevention efforts, which could effectively cut the number of individuals with cancer to begin with. Critics of the cancer community like Samuel Epstein and Moss make this a cornerstone of their critique of the National Cancer Institute and others; there is a certain amount of truth to it. Although efforts to prevent skin cancer through reduced ultraviolet (UV) exposure have increased along with other means of prevention, there is still a short-changing in terms of funding that is happening for prevention efforts. Reallocating some of those funds from treatment to prevention by the American Cancer Society and the NCI would make it easier for researchers and scientists to pursue different lines of research and not be so influenced by the types of grants and funding available to them.

What keeps doctors and scientists from following through on these recommendations and work to overcome these limitations? For one, it's hard to change what you can't admit or recognize. It is far easier to understand our own individual attitudes and opinions than it is to understand a profession as a whole. Some may be wary of assigning such beliefs to such a wide and diverse group of people; obviously, not all people in the medical or scientific field feel that treatment should be emphasized or that their own lines of research are unaffected by global scientific tides. Even if that is the case, the fact that these patterns exist and are affecting the way in which cancer research is being conducted is a serious and significant hurdle to progress against cancer.

What makes these recommendations even more difficult to accept or put into practice is that to make any sort of difference, they have to be adopted by a large number of people; if only one or two scientists understand this phenomenon and change their research practices, it will not change the way in which grant money is sought after or that successful research publications are considered for prestige and promotion in academic fields. It is the very essence of the collective action problem described in Chapter 6. There is no motivation for just a few individuals to undertake the hard work of carrying out change unless it will be adopted by the whole. It would also have to involve quite a bit of soul searching by the medical and scientific community as a whole, something they may be unwilling to do.

The best we can hope for, then, is perhaps that a small minority of scientists and doctors have the ability to pursue the research where it sends them, to be able to tackle questions because they are interesting, intriguing, and important, not because they are the ones that are most likely to be published or received funding. It is often difficult for more radical ideas or approaches to take hold, sometimes because they lack credibility, like the cases of Laetrile or vitamin C. But at some point, all treatments could have been considered radical except for a group of scientists who adopted and pursued them regardless of cost.

The Patients

It's hard to imagine that in the most horrible of times, those moments when people are told they have cancer and they contemplate the future, that the thought of politics should enter into their mind. Surely, there are far more important things for them to worry about—the course of treatment, the odds of survival, the effects on their families. Unfortunately, as this book has detailed, politics permeates most aspects of cancer medicine and treatment, from the drugs that are available to be used and the drug trials used to test them, to the very types of research that doctors are pursuing. It would be pointless to ask cancer patients to try to learn and understand not only about their disease but the politics of it as well. Instead, the best lesson that can be learned is for a patient and their family to be their own best advocate, to search out the most cutting-edge technologies and trials, to ask questions, and more importantly, to ask the right questions.

These suggestions are all commonplace ones that cancer patients often hear. But added to this list would be to become involved in the political process as well. Even though cancer and its related issues are not usually discussed on the campaign trail or by elected officials, patients, and citizens as well, should thoroughly understand how their representatives feel about research funding and support for the various bureaucracies in charge of carrying out cancer policies. This is certainly not to say or imply that one party or the other is more amenable to supporting relevant policies; not every Republican supports every Republican principle and not every Democrat supports every Democratic principle. Nor is it to say that citizens should become single-issue voters, casting a ballot only for those who are most supportive of the fight against cancer. Instead, it is to suggest that patients, along with the rest of us, understand the full realm of policies which our government is concerned with and involved in.

Far too often in this country, people either forget to vote or care not to or change the channel from the nightly news, instead preferring something more entertaining to watch. The news is often hard to digest and politics even harder to comprehend. Despite these hurdles, those who are most affected by policy must either continue to be involved in politics or ensure their participation in the future. The best part is that voting is not the only way to do this; there are multiple ways of participating in politics, including writing letters (or e-mails today), volunteering, and even becoming involved in interest groups like the American Cancer Society. Based on the findings particularly of Chapter 6, participating in interest groups like the ACS may be the most influential action of all. Although their lobbying force is sizeable, it still pales in comparison to the efforts of the AMA and the pharmaceutical industry. Active participation in interest groups spreads out the costs of action and magnifies the efforts of all those involved. A classic example of this phenomenon is that of gun rights and the National Rifle Association. Seeing the issue of gun control, gun rights, and the Second Amendment as vital to their American life, the members of the NRA comprise a political force that, when used effectively and practically in unison, has had a significant effect in policy making. Imagine if the ACS could create a political force for cancer akin to the NRA's support for gun rights; if the ACS could coordinate members' efforts to vote for specific candidates and lobby Congress on particular bills, we could quickly see changes in cancer policy. This goes not only for cancer patients and their families but every citizen in America. If everyone in the policy game is playing according to their selfish motivations, surely cancer patients can do the same. Indeed, they perhaps have the most selfish reason of all to participate—life.

One historical model for such action is activism of the HIV/AIDS community in the 1980s and 1990s. As the epidemic became greater and greater and more strain was placed on the gay and lesbian communities in both California and New York, organizations like ACT UP (the AIDS Coalition to Unleash Power) gathered in New York City, bringing together not only LGBT community members but those involved in AIDS activism. As a group, they were able to harness their anger and frustration in a coordinated movement that was able to force agencies like the NIH, the CDC, and the FDA to place a greater emphasis on AIDS research and medications. In fact, much of this early LGBT organizing and activism have helped lead to wider policy gains such as marriage equality and civil rights for LGBTQ individuals. This is not to say that the comparison between HIV/AIDS activism and cancer is complete; certainly, the two diseases are quite different in their history, their outcomes, and the groups that are likely to suffer from them. However, there are many similarities in knowledge and research barriers along with similar criticisms that could be levied at the FDA and NIH for not doing enough to focus on such issues. The bottom line is that activists involved with ACT UP and other groups were able to not only coalesce but realize the significant impact that government had in their disease and their suffering and organize to do something about it.

Perhaps a better model would be the one detailed by Phil Brown and Edwin J. Mikkelsen in *No Safe Place: Toxic Waste, Leukemia, and Community Action*. Brown and Mikkelsen explore a cluster of childhood leukemia cases in the 1970s and 1980s in the Boston suburb of Woburn; this cluster would eventually be tied to water wells polluted with industrial waste. Unfortunately, the Woburn cluster was not discovered by public health officials or even the EPA, but the parents and community members themselves in a process Brown and Mikkelsen call "popular epidemiology." Before they could garner any attention to draw allies to their fight, the families first had to become activists and

> [t]o become activists, citizens must overcome an ingrained reluctance to challenge authority: they must shed their preconceptions about the role and function of government and about democratic participation. They must also develop a new outlook on the nature of scientific inquiry and the participation of the public in scientific controversy. Activists must learn how to mobilize and organize the public to challenge government successfully. Most of all, as the affected families and other activists in Woburn discovered, enormous patience and energy are required, because the struggle can continue for more than a decade.[1]

The Woburn families and community formed an organization called For a Cleaner Environment, or FACE, in order to understand the origins of the leukemia cluster and to fight for solutions to it. While FACE was eventually able to draw the attention of researchers, allies, and government officials, their most significant action was to sue the two companies accused of polluting the groundwater.

One major difference between the Woburn case and many other cancer cases is the environmental link to the disease. As we have detailed throughout, many scientists, doctors, and government officials are dubious about environmental causes of cancer for many reasons, the least of which would be the assignation of blame for the causing of a disease. However, as more and more scientists come to understand environmental and upstream causes of cancer, popular epidemiology, or the public participation in scientific processes, can shine a light on cancer clusters and provide an example for the organization of patient communities to combat cancer.

One of the possible solutions that Woburn citizens faced in fighting back was simply to leave the community, to leave the area that was causing so much harm. However, one of the most striking findings that Brown and Mikkelsen found was the contention among residents that there was no safe place anywhere; if environmental pollution could be anywhere, then there is nowhere anyone can go to truly feel like they live in a safe and healthy location. Given the possible environmental causes and the fact that everyone is susceptible to cancer, the same can be said of all of us. There is no safe place to hide from cancer. There is no place to go to feel like we can escape it. The only hope we have is in fighting it. Activism on the part of patients and the wider community is potentially very powerful, as Woburn, HIV/AIDS, and even the breast cancer movement have shown us. However, activism is also practically limited; the many hurdles detailed by Brown and Mikkelsen must be overcome along with government and scientific inertia to continue along as it has always been. This ultimately puts the community and potential activists at a severe disadvantage. And if there is no safe place from cancer, this is an issue that affects every single one of us, making us all potential activists. Becoming knowledgeable, concerned, and interested can make us not only activists but participant-scientists in the fight against cancer.

Notes

Chapter One

1. Siddhartha Mukherjee. *The Emperor of All Maladies: A Biography of Cancer* (New York: Scribner, 2010).

2. Ibid., 82.

3. Ibid., 88.

4. R.F. Bud, "Strategy in American Cancer Research After World War II: A Case Study," *Social Studies of Science* 8, no. 4 (1978): 425–59.

5. Siddhartha Mukherjee. *The Emperor of All Maladies: A Biography of Cancer* (New York: Scribner, 2010).

6. Ibid.

7. Ibid., 280.

8. Ibid., 277–278.

9. Phil Brown, Sabrina McCormick, Brian Mayer, Stephen Zavestoski, Rachel Morello-Forsch, Rebecca Gasior Altman, and Laura Senier, "'A Lab of Our Own': Environmental Causation of Breast Cancer and Challenges to the Dominant Epidemiological Paradigm," *Science, Technology, and Human Values* 31, no. 5 (2006): 513.

10. Robert N. Proctor. *Cancer Wars: How Politics Shapes What We Know and Don't Know About Cancer* (New York: Basic Books, 1995).

11. Ibid.

12. Ibid.; Samuel S. Epstein, *The Politics of Cancer Revisited* (New York: East Ridge Press, 1998).

13. David Nathan and Edward J. Benz, "Comprehensive Cancer Centres and the War on Cancer," *Nature Reviews: Cancer* 1, December (2001): 240–45.

Christine Merenda, "How Far Has the War on Cancer Come in the Past 40 Years?," *ONS Connect* June (2012): 20.

14. Christine Merenda, "How Far Has the War on Cancer Come in the Past 40 Years?," *ONS Connect* June (2012): 20.

15. Devra Davis, *The Secret History of the War on Cancer* (New York: Basic Books, 2007: 276).

16. Salvador Luria, "Reflections on Democracy, Science, and Cancer," *Bulletin of the American Academy of Arts and Sciences* 30, no. 5 (1977): 21.

17. Woodrow Wilson, "The Study of Administration," *Political Science Quarterly* 2, no. 2 (1887): 197–222.

18. Ibid., 197.

19. American Association for the Advancement of Science, "Historical Trends in Federal R&D," *AAAS.org*, accessed May 23, 2016 http://www.aaas.org/page/historical-trends-federal-rd.

20. Ibid.

21. Gerald Kutcher, "Cancer Therapy and Military Cold-War Research: Crossing Epistemological and Ethical Boundaries," *History Workshop Journal* 56, Autumn (2003): 105–30.

22. Ibid.

23. Richard Severo, "William Proxmire, Maverick Senator from Wisconsin, Is Dead at 90," *New York Times*, published December 16, 2005, accessed May 23, 2016 http://www.nytimes.com/2005/12/16/us/william-proxmire-maverick-democratic-senator-from-wisconsin-is-dead-at-90.html.

24. John Sides, "Why Congress Should Not Cut Funding to the Social Sciences," *The Washington Post Monkey Cage*, published 2015, accessed May 23, 2016 https://www.washingtonpost.com/blogs/monkey-cage/wp/2015/06/10/why-congress-should-not-cut-funding-to-the-social-sciences/.

25. David Mayhew, *Congress: The Electoral Connection* (New Haven: Yale UP, 1974).

26. Phil Brown, Sabrina McCormick, Brian Mayer, Stephen Zavestoski, Rachel Morello-Forsch, Rebecca Gasior Altman, and Laura Senier, "'A Lab of Our Own': Environmental Causation of Breast Cancer and Challenges to the Dominant Epidemiological Paradigm," *Science, Technology, and Human Values* 31, no. 5 (2006): 505.

27. Sheila Jasanoff, "Science, Politics, and the Renegotiation of Expertise at EPA," *Osiris* 7, Science after '40 (1992): 203.

28. Open Science Collaboration, "Estimating the Reproducibility of Psychological Science," *Science* 349, no. 4716 (2015): 943–951.

29. Brendan Gillespie, Dave Eva, and Ron Johnston, "Carcinogenic Risk Assessment in the United States and Great Britain: The Case of Aldrin/Dieldrin," *Social Studies of Science* 9, no. 3 (1979): 265–301.

30. Ibid.

31. Samuel S. Epstein, *The Politics of Cancer Revisited* (New York: East Ridge Press, 1998).

32. Ibid.

33. John Abraham and Rachel Ballinger, "The Neoliberal Regulatory State, Industry Interest, and the Ideological Penetration of Scientific Knowledge: Deconstructing the Redefinition of Carcinogens in Pharmaceuticals," *Science, Technology, & Human Values* 37, no. 5 (2012): 443–77.

34. Ibid.

35. Evelleen Richards, "The Politics of Therapeutic Evaluation: The Vitamin C and Cancer Controversy," *Social Studies of Science* 18, no. 4 (1988): 653–701.

36. Ibid.

37. Ibid.

38. Ibid., 669.

39. Phil Brown, Sabrina McCormick, Brian Mayer, Stephen Zavestoski, Rachel Morello-Forsch, Rebecca Gasior Altman, and Laura Senier, "'A Lab of Our Own': Environmental Causation of Breast Cancer and Challenges to the Dominant Epidemiological Paradigm," *Science, Technology, and Human Values* 31, no. 5 (2006): 505.

40. Ibid., 507.

41. Ibid.

42. Frances B. McCrea and Gerald E. Markle, "The Estrogen Replacement Controversy in the USA and UL: Different Answers to the Same Question?" *Social Studies of Science* 14, no. 1 (1984): 15.

43. Ibid.

44. Thomas H. Murray, "Regulating Asbestos: Ethics, Politics, and Scientific Values," *Science, Technology, & Human Values* 11, no. 3 (1986): 1.

45. Brianna Rego, "The Polonium Brief: A Hidden History of Cancer, Radiation, and the Tobacco Industry," *Isis* 100, no. 3 (2009), 453.

46. Mark Parascandola, "Uncertain Science and a Failure of Trust: The NIH Radioepidemiologic Tables and Compensation for Radiation-Induced Cancer," *Isis* 93, no. 4 (2002): 456.

47. Ibid.

48. Sheila Jasanoff, "American Exceptionalism and the Political Acknowledgement of Risk," *Daedalus* 119, no. 4 (1990): 61–81.

49. Sabrina McCormick, "Democratizing Science Movements: A New Framework for Mobilization and Contestation," *Social Studies of Science* 37, no. 4 (2007): 609.

50. Harvey M. Sapolsky, "The Politics of Risk," *Daedalus* 119, no. 4 (1990): 83–96.

51. James C. Petersen and Gerald E. Markle, "Politics and Science in the Laetrile Controversy," *Social Studies of Science* 9, no. 2 (1979): 139–66.

52. Ibid.

53. Ibid., 150.

54. Ibid.

55. Neil Gross, *Why Are Professors Liberal and Why Do Conservatives Care?* (Cambridge, MA: Harvard UP, 2013).

56. Sheila Jasanoff, "American Exceptionalism and the Political Acknowledgement of Risk," *Daedalus* 119, no. 4 (1990): 61–81.

Sheila Jasanoff, "Science, Politics, and the Renegotiation of Expertise at EPA," *Osiris* 7, Science after '40 (1992): 203.

57. Sheila Jasanoff, "American Exceptionalism and the Political Acknowledgement of Risk," *Daedalus* 119, no. 4 (1990): 61–81.

58. Harvey M. Sapolsky, "The Politics of Risk," *Daedalus* 119, no. 4 (1990): 83.

59. Barry R. Weingast and Mark J. Moran, "Bureaucratic Discretion or Congressional Control? Regulatory Policymaking by the Federal Trade Commission," *The Journal of Political Economy* 91, no. 5 (1983): 765–800.

Terry M. Moe, "Control and Feedback in Economic Regulation: The Case of the NLRB," *American Political Science Review* 79, no. 4 (1985): 1095–16.

B. Dan Wood and Richard W. Waterman, "The Dynamics of Political Control of the Bureaucracy," *American Political Science Review* 85, no. 3 (1991): 801–28.

Marissa Martino Golden, *What Motivates Bureaucrats? Politics and Administration During the Reagan Years* (New York: Columbia UP, 2000).

David Hedge and Renee J. Johnson, "The Plot that Failed: The Republican Revolution and Congressional Control of the Bureaucracy," *JPART* 12, no. 3 (2002): 333–51.

60. W.D. Kay, *Can Democracies Fly in Space? The Challenge of Revitalizing the U.S. Space Program* (Westport, CT: Praeger, 1995).

Chapter Two

1. American Cancer Society, "Where Does Your Money Go?," *Cancer.org*, accessed May 27, 2016 http://www.cancer.org/research/infographicgallery/where-does-money-go-2015.

2. Margaret I. Cuomo, *A World Without Cancer: The Making of a New Cure and the Real Promise of Prevention* (New York: Rodale, 2012).

3. Ibid.

National Cancer Institute, "2013 Fact Book," *Cancer.gov*, published 2013, accessed May 27, 2016 at http://www.cancer.gov/aboutnci/budget_planning_leg/fact-book-2013.

4. Samuel S. Epstein, *The Politics of Cancer Revisited* (New York: East Ridge Press, 1998).

Robert N. Proctor, *Cancer Wars: How Politics Shapes What We Know and Don't Know About Cancer* (New York: Basic Books, 1995).

David Nathan and Edward J. Benz, "Comprehensive Cancer Centres and the War on Cancer," *Nature Reviews: Cancer* 1, December (2001): 240–245.

Devra Davis, *The Secret History of the War on Cancer* (New York: Basic Books, 2007).

Christine Merenda, "How Far Has the War on Cancer Come in the Past 40 Years?" *ONS Connect* June (2012): 20.

5. Samuel S. Epstein, *The Politics of Cancer Revisited* (New York: East Ridge Press, 1998), 334.

6. Robert N. Proctor, *Cancer Wars: How Politics Shapes What We Know and Don't Know About Cancer* (New York: Basic Books, 1995).

7. Wendy Whitman Cobb, "Who's Supporting Space Activities? An 'Issue Public' for US Space Policy," *Space Policy* 27, no. 4 (2011): 234–39.

8. American Association for the Advancement of Science, "Historical Trends in Federal R&D," *AAAS.org*, published 2016, accessed May 23, 2016 at http://www.aaas.org/page/historical-trends-federal-rd.

9. Barry R. Weingast and Mark J. Moran, "Bureaucratic Discretion or Congressional Control? Regulatory Policymaking by the Federal Trade Commission," *The Journal of Political Economy* 91, no. 5 (1983): 765–800.

Terry M. Moe, "Control and Feedback in Economic Regulation: The Case of the NLRB," *American Political Science Review* 79, no. 4 (1985): 1095–116.

B. Dan Wood and Richard W. Waterman, "The Dynamics of Political Control of the Bureaucracy," *American Political Science Review* 85, no. 3 (1991): 801–28.

Marissa Martino Golden, *What Motivates Bureaucrats? Politics and Administration During the Reagan Years* (New York: Columbia UP, 2000).

David Hedge and Renee J. Johnson, "The Plot that Failed: The Republican Revolution and Congressional Control of the Bureaucracy," *JPART* 12, no. 3 (2002): 333–51.

10. Barry R. Weingast, Kenneth A. Shepsle, and Christopher Johnsen, "The Political Economy of Benefits and Costs: A Neoclassical Approach to Distributive Politics," *Journal of Political Economy* 89, no. 4 (1981): 643.

11. Robert M. Stein and Kenneth N. Bickers, "Universalism and the Electoral Connection: A Test and Some Doubts," *Political Research Quarterly* 47, no. 2 (1994): 295–96.

12. David Mayhew, *Congress: The Electoral Connection* (New Haven: Yale UP, 1974).

13. The confusion among the terms appears to extend to researchers themselves. In two papers published practically simultaneously, Stein and Bickers use the term "universalism" in the title of one and the term "pork barrel" in the title of the other.

14. Robert M. Stein and Kenneth N. Bickers, "Universalism and the Electoral Connection: A Test and Some Doubts," *Political Research Quarterly* 47, no. 2 (1994): 295–96.

Robert M. Stein and Kenneth N. Bickers, "Congressional Elections and the Pork Barrel," *The Journal of Politics*, 56, no. 2 (1994): 377–99.

15. Barry R. Weingast, "Reflections on Distributive Politics and Universalism," *Political Research Quarterly*, 47, no. 2 (1994): 319–27.

16. David G. Smith, "Federal Health Grants and Regional Health Politics," *Publius* 12, no. 2 (1982): 63–77.

Michael Mintrom, "Competitive Federalism and the Governance of Controversial Science," *Publius* 39, no. 4 (2009): 606–31.

Vincent T. DeVita and Elizabeth DeVita-Raeburn. *The Death of Cancer* (New York: Sarah Crichton Books, 2015).

17. David G. Smith, "Federal Health Grants and Regional Health Politics," *Publius* 12, no. 2 (1982): 63–77.

18. Michael Mintrom, "Competitive Federalism and the Governance of Controversial Science," *Publius* 39, no. 4 (2009): 606–31.

19. David G. Smith, "Federal Health Grants and Regional Health Politics," *Publius* 12, no. 2 (1982): 63–77.

20. Rick K. Wilson, "An Empirical Test of Preferences for the Political Pork Barrel: District Level Appropriations for River and Harbor Legislation, 1889–1913," *American Journal of Political Science* 30, no. 4 (1986): 729–754.

David P. Baron, "Distributive Politics and the Persistence of Amtrak," *The Journal of Politics* 52, no. 3 (1990): 883–913.

21. Robert M. Stein and Kenneth N. Bickers, "Universalism and the Electoral Connection: A Test and Some Doubts," *Political Research Quarterly* 47, no. 2 (1994): 295–96.

Emerson M.S. Niou and Peter C. Ordeshook, "Universalism in Congress," *American Journal of Political Science* 29, no. 2 (1985): 246–58.

22. Oskar Nupia, "Distributive Politics, Number of Parties, Ideological Polarization, and Bargaining Power," *The Journal of Politics* 75, no. 2 (2013): 410–21.

23. Robert A. Dahl and Charles Lindblom, *Politics, Economics, and Welfare* (New York: Harper and Row, 1953).

Charles Lindblom, "The Science of Muddling Through," *Public Administration Review* 19 (1959): 79–88.

Aaron Wildavsky, *The Politics of the Budgetary Process* (Boston: Little Brown, 1964).

Otto A. Davis, M.A.H. Dempster, and Aaron Wildavsky, "A Theory of the Budgetary Process," *American Political Science Review* 60 (1966): 529–47.

24. William D. Berry, "The Confusing Case of Budgetary Incrementalism: Too Many Meanings for a Single Concept," *The Journal of Politics* 52, no. 1 (1990): 167–96.

25. Ibid.

26. Kathleen Peroff and Margaret Podolak-Warren, "Does Spending on Defence Cut Spending on Health? A Time Series Analysis of the US Economy, 1929–74," *British Journal of Political Science* 9, no. 1 (1979): 21–39.

27. Wendy N. Whitman Cobb, *Unbroken Government: Success and the Illusion of Failure in Policymaking* (New York: Palgrave Macmillan, 2013).

28. Thomas A. Birkland, "Focusing Events, Mobilization, and Agenda Setting," *Journal of Public Policy* 18, no. 1 (1998): 53–74.

29. R.F. Bud, "Strategy in American Cancer Research After World War II: A Case Study," *Social Studies of Science* 8, no. 4 (1978): 425–59.

30. Martin L. Brown and Arnold L. Potosky, "The Presidential Effect: The Public Health Response to Media Coverage About Ronald Reagan's Colon Cancer Episode," *The Public Opinion Quarterly* 54, no. 3 (1990): 317–29.

Vincent Price, et al., "Locating the Issue Public: The Multi-Dimensional Nature of Engagement with Health Care Reform," *Political Behavior* 28, no. 1 (2006): 33–63.

David W. Brady and Daniel P. Kessler, "Who Supports Health Reform?" *PS: Political Science and Politics* 43, no. 1 (2010): 1–6.

Andrew Karch, "Vertical Diffusion and the Policymaking Process: The Politics of Embryonic Stem Cell Research," *Political Research Quarterly* 65, no. 1 (2012): 48–61.

31. Joe Stork, "Political Aspects of Health," *Middle East Report* 161 (1989): 4–10.

32. Samuel S. Epstein, et al., "The Crisis in US and International Cancer Policy," *The Politics of Scientific Research* 32, no. 4 (2002): 669–707.

33. American Cancer Society, "Where Does Your Money Go?" Cancer.org, accessed 14 December 2016 at http://www.cancer.org/research/infographicgallery/where-does-money-go-2016

34. Devra Davis, *The Secret History of the War on Cancer* (New York: Basic Books, 2007).

35. Maureen Hogan Casamayou, *The Politics of Breast Cancer* (Washington, D.C.: Georgetown UP, 2001).

36. Harvey M. Sapolsky, "The Politics of Risk," *Daedalus* 119, no. 4 (1990): 94.

37. Mark E. Rushefsky, *Making Cancer Policy* (Albany: SUNY Press, 1986).

38. Ibid.

39. Lisa A. Bero, et al. "Science in Regulatory Policy Making: Case Studies in the Development of Workplace Smoking Restrictions," *Tobacco Control* 10, no. 4 (2001): 329–36.

40. Samuel S. Epstein, *The Politics of Cancer Revisited* (New York: East Ridge Press, 1998).

41. Robert N. Proctor, *Cancer Wars: How Politics Shapes What We Know and Don't Know About Cancer* (New York: Basic Books, 1995).

42. Ralph W. Moss, *The Cancer Industry* (Brooklyn: Equinox Press, 1996: 11).

43. Hagop Kantarjian, et al., "High Cancer Drug Prices in the United States: Reasons and Proposed Solutions," *Journal of Oncology Practice* 10, no. 4 (2014): 208–11.

Mustaqueem Siddiqui and S. Vincent Rajkumar, "The High Cost of Cancer Drugs and What We Can Do About It," *Mayo Clinic Proceedings* 87, no. 10 (2012): 935–43.

David H. Howard, et al., "Pricing in the Market for Anticancer Drugs," *Journal of Economic Perspectives* 29, no. 1 (2015): 139–62.

44. National Cancer Institute, "Cancer Costs Projected to Reach at Least $158 Billion in 2020," *Cancer.gov*, published 2011, accessed May 27, 2016 at http://www.cancer.gov/news-events/press-releases/2011/CostCancer2020.

45. Devra Davis, *The Secret History of the War on Cancer* (New York: Basic Books, 2007).

46. Richard S. Conley and Wendy Whitman Cobb, "Presidential Vision or Congressional Derision? Explaining Budgeting Outcomes for NASA, 1958–2008," *Congress and the Presidency* 39, no. 1 (2012): 51–73.

47. This pattern of unanimity or near-unanimity in passing cancer legislation can also be interpreted as evidence for the distributive nature of cancer funding. Shepsle and Weingast (1981, 96) note that pork barrel politics is "characterized by legislative support coalitions well in excess of minimal winning size and often approaching unanimous size."

48. David G. Smith, "Federal Health Grants and Regional Health Politics," *Publius* 12, no. 2 (1982): 63–77.

49. Kathleen Peroff and Margaret Podolak-Warren, "Does Spending on Defence Cut Spending on Health? A Time Series Analysis of the US Economy, 1929–74," *British Journal of Political Science* 9, no. 1 (1979): 21–39.

50. The number of Republicans could have been easily substituted. The variable is simply used as an indicator of chamber ideology—the more Democrats there are, the more theoretically liberal the chamber should be.

51. Wendy N. Whitman Cobb, *Unbroken Government: Success and the Illusion of Failure in Policymaking* (New York: Palgrave Macmillan, 2013).

52. Joe Stork, "Political Aspects of Health," *Middle East Report* 161 (1989): 4–10.

53. Maureen Hogan Casamayou, *The Politics of Breast Cancer* (Washington, D.C.: Georgetown UP, 2001).

54. Joe Stork, "Political Aspects of Health," *Middle East Report* 161 (1989): 4.

Chapter Three

1. David Nathan and Edward J. Benz, "Comprehensive Cancer Centres and the War on Cancer," *Nature Reviews: Cancer* 1, December (2001): 243.

2. Joe Biden, "Inspiring a New Generation to Defy the Bounds of Innovation: A Moonshot to Cure Cancer," *Medium*, published January 12 2016, accessed 13 January 2016 https://medium.com/cancer-moonshot/inspiring-a-new-generation -to-defy-the-bounds-of-innovation-a-moonshot-to-cure-cancer-fbdf71d01c2e# .2ayjn8jk2.

3. Samuel Kernell, *Going Public: New Strategies of Presidential Leadership Fourth Edition* (Washington, D.C.: CQ Press, 2006).

4. Joe Biden, "Inspiring a New Generation to Defy the Bounds of Innovation: A Moonshot to Cure Cancer," *Medium*, published January 12, 2016, accessed 13 January 2016 https://medium.com/cancer-moonshot/inspiring-a-new-generation -to-defy-the-bounds-of-innovation-a-moonshot-to-cure-cancer-fbdf71d01c2e# .2ayjn8jk2.

5. Samuel S. Epstein, *The Politics of Cancer Revisited* (New York: East Ridge Press, 1998).

6. Ibid., 363–64.

7. National Cancer Institute, "Step 4: NCI Funding Determinations," *Cancer .gov*, published 2015, accessed June 12, 2016 http://www.cancer.gov/grants-training /grants-process/application/funding.

8. Barry R. Weingast and Mark J. Moran, "Bureaucratic Discretion or Congressional Control? Regulatory Policymaking by the Federal Trade Commission," *The Journal of Political Economy* 91, no. 5 (1983): 765–800.

Terry M. Moe, "Control and Feedback in Economic Regulation: The Case of the NLRB," *American Political Science Review* 79, no. 4 (1985): 1095–1116.

B. Dan Wood and Richard W. Waterman, "The Dynamics of Political Control of the Bureaucracy," *American Political Science Review* 85, no. 3 (1991): 801–28.

Marissa Martino Golden, *What Motivates Bureaucrats? Politics and Administration During the Reagan Years* (New York: Columbia UP, 2000).

David Hedge and Renee J. Johnson, "The Plot that Failed: The Republican Revolution and Congressional Control of the Bureaucracy," *JPART* 12, no. 3 (2002): 333–51.

9. Jason A. MacDonald, "Limitation Riders and Congressional Influence over Bureaucratic Policy Decisions," *American Political Science Review* 104, no. 4 (2010): 766–82.

10. Sheila Jasanoff, *The Fifth Branch: Science Advisors as Policymakers* (Cambridge, MA: Harvard UP, 1990).

11. Ibid., 66.

12. Mark E. Rushefsky, *Making Cancer Policy* (Albany: SUNY Press, 1986).

13. Sheila Jasanoff, *The Fifth Branch: Science Advisors as Policymakers* (Cambridge, MA: Harvard UP, 1990).

14. Ibid., 85.

15. Ibid., 87.

16. Marieka S. Schotland and Lisa A. Bero, "Evaluating Public Commentary and Scientific Evidence Submitted in the Development of a Risk Assessment," *Risk Analysis* 22 no. 1 (2002): 131–40.

Lisa A. Bero, Theresa Montini, Katherine Bryan-Jones, and Christina Mangurian, "Science in Regulatory Policy Making: Case Studies in the Development of Workplace Smoking Restrictions," *Tobacco Control* 10, no. 4 (2001): 329–36.

17. Sheila Jasanoff, *The Fifth Branch: Science Advisors as Policymakers* (Cambridge, MA: Harvard UP, 1990).

Sheila Jasanoff, "American Exceptionalism and the Political Acknowledgement of Risk," *Daedalus* 119, no. 4 (1990): 61–81.

18. Richard A. Merrill, "Food Safety Regulation: Reforming the Delaney Clause," *Annual Review of Public Health* 18 (1997): 315.

19. Ibid.

20. Daniel Carpenter, *Reputation and Power: Organizational Image and Pharmaceutical Regulation at the FDA* (Princeton, NJ: Princeton UP, 2010).

21. Department of Health and Human Services, "Food and Drug Administration: Justification of Estimates for Appropriations Committees," *FDA.gov*, accessed June 28, 2016 http://www.fda.gov/downloads/AboutFDA/ReportsManualsForms/Reports/BudgetReports/UCM388309.pdf.

22. Daniel Carpenter, *Reputation and Power: Organizational Image and Pharmaceutical Regulation at the FDA* (Princeton, NJ: Princeton UP, 2010).

23. Ibid.

John Abraham, "Scientific Standards and Institutional Interests: Carcinogenic Risk Assessment of Benoxaprofen in the UK and the US," *Social Studies of Science* 23, no. 3 (1993): 387–444.

Sheila Jasanoff, *The Fifth Branch: Science Advisors as Policymakers* (Cambridge, MA: Harvard UP, 1990).

Harvey M. Sapolsky, "The Politics of Risk," *Daedalus* 119, no. 4 (1990): 83–96.

24. Daniel Carpenter, *Reputation and Power: Organizational Image and Pharmaceutical Regulation at the FDA* (Princeton, NJ: Princeton UP, 2010).

25. Chul Kim and Vinay Prasad, "Strength of Validation for Surrogate End Points Used in the US Food and Drug Administration's Approval of Oncology Drugs," *Mayo Clinic Proceedings* 91 no. 6 (2016): 713–25.

Sy Mukherjee, "Cancer Drugs Are the Least Likely to Receive FDA Approval," *Fortune.com*, published 2016, accessed June 28, 2016 http://fortune.com/2016/05/26/drugs-most-likely-to-be-approved/.

26. Chul Kim and Vinay Prasad, "Strength of Validation for Surrogate End Points Used in the US Food and Drug Administration's Approval of Oncology Drugs," *Mayo Clinic Proceedings* 91 no. 6 (2016): 713–25.

27. Daniel Carpenter, *Reputation and Power: Organizational Image and Pharmaceutical Regulation at the FDA* Princeton, NJ: Princeton UP, 2010), 496–97.

28. Sy Mukherjee, "Cancer Drugs Are the Least Likely to Receive FDA Approval," *Fortune.com*, published 2016, accessed June 28, 2016 http://fortune.com/2016/05/26/drugs-most-likely-to-be-approved/.

29. Daniel Carpenter, *Reputation and Power: Organizational Image and Pharmaceutical Regulation at the FDA* (Princeton, NJ: Princeton UP, 2010).

30. Helena Bottemiller Evich, "Former Commissioners: Make FDA An Independent Agency," *Politico*, published June 25, 2016, accessed July 2, 2016 http://www.politico.com/story/2016/06/former-commissioners-make-fda-a-cabinet-level-agency-224803.

31. Daniel Carpenter, *Reputation and Power: Organizational Image and Pharmaceutical Regulation at the FDA* (Princeton, NJ: Princeton UP, 2010), 515.

32. S. Vincent Rajkumar, "Drug Approvals in Oncology: Striking the Right Balance Between Saving Lives and Patient Safety," *Mayo Clinic Proceedings* 91, no. 6 (2016): 689–91.

33. Daniel Carpenter, *Reputation and Power: Organizational Image and Pharmaceutical Regulation at the FDA* (Princeton, NJ: Princeton UP, 2010), 515.

34. Ibid.

35. Ibid.

36. Daniel Carpenter, *Reputation and Power: Organizational Image and Pharmaceutical Regulation at the FDA* (Princeton, NJ: Princeton UP, 2010), 473.

37. Ibid.

38. Ibid., 476.

39. Ibid., 303.

40. Sheila Jasanoff, *The Fifth Branch: Science Advisors as Policymakers* (Cambridge, MA: Harvard UP, 1990).

41. Daniel Carpenter, *Reputation and Power: Organizational Image and Pharmaceutical Regulation at the FDA* (Princeton, NJ: Princeton UP, 2010), 201.

42. Ibid.

43. Ibid., 206.

44. While an enhanced quantitative examination using linear or logistic regression was considered, the N in this case is too small (20) to allow for any significant conclusions to be drawn.

45. David Hedge and Renee J. Johnson, "The Plot that Failed: The Republican Revolution and Congressional Control of the Bureaucracy," *JPART* 12, no. 3 (2002): 333–51.

Chapter Four

1. Richard E. Neustadt, *Presidential Power and the Modern Presidents: The Politics of Leadership from Roosevelt to Reagan* (New York: The Free Press, 1990), 11.

2. George Bush, "Interviews with NBC Owned and Operated Television Stations," *The American Presidency Project*, editors Gerhard Peters and John T. Woolley, published November 20, 1991, accessed July 7, 2015 http://presidency.ucsb.edu/ws/?pid=20249.

3. William J. Clinton, "Remarks in Knoxville, Tennessee," *The American Presidency Project*, editors Gerhard Peters and John T. Woolley, published October 10, 1996, accessed July 7, 2016 http://www.presidency.ucsb.edu/ws/?pid=52079.

4. William Howard Taft, "Special Message, April 9, 1910," *The American Presidency Project*, editors Gerhard Peters and John T. Woolley, published April 9, 1910, accessed July 8, 2016 http://www.presidency.ucsb.edu/ws/?pid=68499.

5. Herbert Hoover, "Remarks at a Ceremony Honoring Madame Marie Curie, October 30, 1929," *The American Presidency Project*, editors Gerhard Peters and John T. Woolley, published October 30, 1929, accessed July 9, 2016 http://www.presidency.ucsb.edu/ws/?pid=21989.

6. Herbert Hoover, "Message to a Testimonial Dinner Honoring Dr. James Ewing, January 31, 1931," *The American Presidency Project*, editors Gerhard Peters and John T. Woolley, published January 31, 1931, accessed July 9, 2016 http://www.presidency.ucsb.edu/ws/?pid=22921.

7. Franklin D. Roosevelt, "Radio Address for the Fifth Birthday Ball for Crippled Children, January 29, 1938," *The American Presidency Project*, editors Gerhard Peters and John T. Woolley, published January 29, 1938, accessed July 9, 2016 http://www.presidency.ucsb.edu/ws/?pid=15584.

8. Harry S. Truman, "Special Message to Congress Recommending a Comprehensive Health Program, November 19, 1945," *The American Presidency Project*, editors Gerhard Peters and John T. Woolley, published November 19, 1945, accessed July 9, 2016 http://www.presidency.ucsb.edu/ws/?pid=12288.

9. Ibid.

10. George Bush, "Question-and-Answer Session in Grand Rapids, October 29, 1992," *The American Presidency Project*, editors Gerhard Peters and John T. Woolley, published October 29, 1992, accessed July 9, 2016 http://www.presidency.ucsb.edu/ws/?pid=21708.

11. William J. Clinton, "Remarks on the Anticancer Initiative, March 29, 1996," *The American Presidency Project*, editors Gerhard Peters and John T. Woolley, published March 29, 1996, accessed July 9, 2016 http://www.presidency.ucsb.edu/ws/?pid=52605.

12. William J. Clinton, "Remarks Announcing Anticancer Initiatives, October 27, 1996," *The American Presidency Project*, editors Gerhard Peters and John T. Woolley, published October 27, 1996, accessed July 9, 2016 http://www.presidency.ucsb.edu/ws/?pid=52170.

13. Barack Obama, "Remarks on Health Care Reform, September 10, 2009," *The American Presidency Project*, editors Gerhard Peters and John T. Woolley, published September 10, 2009, accessed July 9, 2016 http://www.presidency.ucsb.edu/ws/?pid=86605.

14. Joe Biden, "Inspiring a New Generation to Defy the Bounds of Innovation: A Moonshot to Cure Cancer," *Medium*, published January 12, 2016, accessed January 13, 2016 https://medium.com/cancer-moonshot/inspiring-a-new-generation-to-defy-the-bounds-of-innovation-a-moonshot-to-cure-cancer-fbdf71d01c2e#.2ayjn8jk2.

15. Maggie Fox, "Cancer 'Moonshot' Plan Aims to Share Information to Speed Fight for Cure," *NBC News*, published June 30, 2016, accessed July 9, 2016 http://www.nbcnews.com/health/cancer/cancer-moonshot-plan-aims-share-information-speed-fight-cure-n601231.

16. Lyndon B. Johnson, "Remarks at the Launching of the 1966 Cancer Crusade, March 31, 1966," *The American Presidency Project*, editors Gerhard Peters and John T. Woolley, published March 31, 1966, accessed July 10, 2016 http://www.presidency.ucsb.edu/ws/?pid=27522.

17. Nancy Gibbs, "Betty Ford, 1918–2011," *Time*, published July 8, 2011, accessed July 10, 2016 http://content.time.com/time/nation/article/0,8599,2082229-3,00.html.

18. Ronald Reagan, "Excerpts from an Interview with Hugh Sidey of Time Magazine, July 25, 1985," *The American Presidency Project*, editors Gerhard Peters and John T. Woolley, published July 25, 1985, accessed July 5, 2016 http://www.presidency.ucsb.edu/ws/?pid=38940.

19. Ibid.

20. Martin L. Brown and Arnold L. Potosky, "The Presidential Effect: The Public Health Response to Media Coverage About Ronald Reagan's Colon Cancer Episode," *The Public Opinion Quarterly* 54, no. 3 (1990): 317–29.

21. John M. Logsdon, *After Apollo? Richard Nixon and the American Space Program* (New York: Palgrave Macmillan, 2015).

22. Ibid.

23. Chuck Shih, Jordan Schwartz, and Allan Coukell, "How Would Government Negotiation of Medicare Part D Drug Prices Work?," *Health Affairs Blog*, posted February 1, 2016, accessed July 11, 2016 http://healthaffairs.org/blog/2016/02/01/how-would-government-negotation-of-medicare-part-d-drug-prices-work/.

Chapter Five

1. David Mayhew, *Congress: The Electoral Connection* (New Haven: Yale UP, 1974), 11.

2. Ibid.

3. *Aid to Physically Handicapped, Part 13: Cancer, United States House of Representatives*, 79th Cong., 1st session (1945) (Committee on Labor).

4. Ibid.

5. *Regional Medical Complexes for Heart Disease, Cancer, Stroke, and Other Diseases, United States House of Representatives*, 89th Cong., 1st session (1965) (Committee on Interstate and Foreign Commerce.

6. *Federal Efforts to Protect the Public from Cancer-Causing Chemicals Are Not Very Effective*, General Accounting Office (1976).

7. *Community-Based Cancer Control Programs, United States House of Representatives*, 96th Cong., 2nd session (1980) (Subcommittee on Oversight and Investigations, Committee on Interstate and Foreign Commerce).

8. *High Prices, Low Transparency: The Bitter Pill of Health Care Costs, United States Senate*, 113th Cong., 1st session (2013) (Committee on Finance).

9. *The Roll Out of HealthCare.gov: The Limitations of Big Government, United State House of Representatives*, 113th Cong., 1st session (2013) (Committee on Oversight and Government Reform).

10. *The Banning of Saccharin, United States Senate*, 95th Cong., 1st session (1977) (Subcommittee on Health and Scientific Research, Committee on Human Resources).

11. *Prostate Cancer, United States Senate*, 106th Cong., 1st session (1999) (Subcommittee of the Committee on Appropriations).

12. *National Cancer Institute's Therapy Program, United States House of Representatives*, 97th Cong., 1st session (1981) (Subcommittee on Health and the Environment, Committee on Energy and Commerce, Subcommittee on Investigations and Oversight, Committee on Science and Technology).

13. Maureen Hogan Casamayou, *The Politics of Breast Cancer* (Washington, D.C.: Georgetown UP, 2001).

14. *Formaldehyde Study, United States House of Representatives*, 99th Cong., 2nd session (1986) (Subcommittee on Oversight and Investigations, Committee on Energy and Commerce). Emphasis added.

15. *Oversight of the National Cancer Institute, 1981, United States Senate*, 97th Cong., 1st session (1981) (Subcommittee on Investigations and General Oversight, Committee on Labor and Human Resources).

16. *Patient Safety and Anticancer Drugs, United States Senate*, 98th Cong., 1st session (1983) (Committee on Labor and Human Resources).

17. Ibid.

18. *Cancer Survival Rates, United States House of Representatives*, 100th Cong., 1st session (1987) (Subcommittee on Health and the Environment, Committee on Energy and Commerce).

19. Ibid., 5.

20. *Scientific and Technical Basis for Radon Policy, United States Senate*, 103rd Cong., 2nd session (1994) (Committee on Energy and Natural Resources).

21. Ibid.

22. *National Cancer Institute's Revision of Its Mammography Guidelines, United States House of Representatives,* 103rd Cong., 2nd session (1994) (Human Resources and Intergovernmental Relations Subcommittee, Committee on Government Operations).

23. Ibid.

24. *Making Sense of the Mammography Controversy: What Women Need to Know, United States Senate*, 107th Cong., 2nd session (2002) (Subcommittee on Public Health of the Committee on Health, Education, Labor, and Pensions, Subcommittee on Labor, Health, and Human Services and Education of the Committee on Appropriations).

25. *Exclusive Agreements Between Federal Agencies and Bristol-Myers Squibb Co. for Drug Development: Is the Public Interest Protected?, United States House of Representatives*, 102nd Cong., 1st session (1991) (Subcommittee on Regulation, Business Opportunities, and Technology, Committee on Small Business).

26. *Pricing of Drugs Codeveloped by Federal Laboratories and Private Companies, United States House of Representatives*, 103rd Cong., 1st session (1993) (Subcommittee on Regulation, Business Opportunities, and Technology, Committee on Small Business).

27. Ibid.

28. Ibid., 10.

29. *Medicare Reimbursement Policies Can Influence the Setting and Cost of Chemotherapy*, General Accounting Office (1992).

30. Vinay Prasad and Sham Mailankody, "The UK Cancer Drugs Fund Experiment and the US Cancer Drug Cost Problem: Bearing the Cost of Cancer Drugs Until It Is Unbearable," *Mayo Clinic Proceedings* 91, no. 6 (2016): 707–12.

Chapter Six

1. American Cancer Society, "Tobacco-Related Cancers Fact Sheet," *Cancer.org*, published February 21, 2014, accessed July 26, 2016 http://www.cancer.org/cancer/cancercauses/tobaccocancer/tobacco-related-cancer-fact-sheet.

2. Ibid.

3. Michael Eriksen, Judith Mackay, Neil Schluger, Farhad Islami Gomeshtapeh, and Jeffrey Drope, *The Tobacco Atlas* (Atlanta, GA: American Cancer Society, 2015).

4. Center for Responsive Politics, "Tobacco Industry Profile, Summary 2015," *Opensecrets.org*, accessed July 26, 2016 http://www.opensecrets.org/lobby/indusclient.php?id=A02&year=2015.

5. Siddhartha Mukherjee, *The Emperor of All Maladies: A Biography of Cancer* (New York: Scribner, 2010).

6. Ibid.

7. American Cancer Society, "Facts About ACS," *Cancer.org*, published April 2015, accessed July 31, 2016 http://www.cancer.org/aboutus/whoweare/acs-fact-sheet.

8. American Cancer Society, "ACS Mission Statements," *Cancer.org*, published November 11, 2008, accessed July 31, 2016 http://www.cancer.org/aboutus/whoweare/acsmissionstatements.

9. Ernst and Young, American Cancer Society, Inc., "Management's Discussion and Analysis and Financial Statements," published 2016, accessed July 31, 2016 http://www.cancer.org/acs/groups/content/@marketing/documents/document/acspc-047908.pdf.

10. Center for Responsive Politics, "American Cancer Society," accessed June 14, 2016 http://www.opensecrets.org/lobby/clientsum.php?id=D000031468&year=2016.

11. Ibid.

12. Ralph W. Moss, *The Cancer Industry* (Brooklyn: Equinox Press, 1996).

13. Ibid., 400.

14. Ibid., 401.

15. Samuel S. Epstein, *The Politics of Cancer Revisited* (New York: East Ridge Press, 1998).

16. Ralph W. Moss, *The Cancer Industry* (Brooklyn: Equinox Press, 1996).

17. Samuel S. Epstein, *The Politics of Cancer Revisited* (New York: East Ridge Press, 1998), 463.

18. Charity Navigator, "American Cancer Society," *CharityNavigator.org*, Published June 1, 2016, accessed July 31, 2016 http://www.charitynavigator.org/index.cfm?bay=search.summary&orgid=6495.

19. Ibid.

20. American Medical Association, "The Founding of the AMA," *AMA-assn.org*, accessed August 1, 2016 http://www.ama-assn.org/ama/pub/about-ama/our-history/the-founding-of-ama.page?.

21. Patricia Ward, "United States versus American Medical Association et al.: The Medical Antitrust Case of 1938–1945," *American Studies* 30, no. 2 (1989): 123–53.

22. Ibid., 130.

23. Rickey Hendricks, "Medical Practice Embattled: Kaiser Permanente, the American Medical Association, Henry J. Kaiser on the West Coast, 1945–1955," *Pacific Historical Review* 60, no. 4 (1991): 439–73.

24. Dan Mangan, "'Pharma Bro' Martin Shkreli Pleads Not Guilty to New Charge," *NBC News*, published June 6, 2016, accessed August 3, 2016 http://www.nbcnews.com/business/business-news/pharma-bro-martin-shkreli-pleads-not-guilty-new-charge-n586676.

25. Peter A. Ubel, Amy P. Abernathy, and S. Yousef Zafar, "Full Disclosure-Out-of-Pocket Costs as Side Effects," *New England Journal of Medicine* 369, no. 16 (2013): 1484–86.

26. Hagop Kantarjian, David Steensma, Judit Rius Sanjuan, Adam Elshaug, and Donald Light, "High Cancer Drug Prices in the United States: Reasons and Proposed Solutions," *Journal of Oncology Practice* 10, no. 4 (2014): 208–11.

27. David H. Howard, Peter B. Back, Ernst R. Berndt, and Rena M. Conti, "Pricing in the Market for Anticancer Drugs," *Journal of Economic Perspectives* 29, no. 1 (2015): 139–62.

28. Hagop Kantarjian, David Steensma, Judit Rius Sanjuan, Adam Elshaug, and Donald Light, "High Cancer Drug Prices in the United States: Reasons and Proposed Solutions," *Journal of Oncology Practice* 10, no. 4 (2014): 208–11.

Mustaqueem Siddiqui and S. Vincent Rajkumar, "The High Cost of Cancer Drugs and What We Can Do About It," *Mayo Clinic Proceedings* 87, no. 10 (2012): 935–43.

29. PhRMA, "Medicines: Cost in Context," *PhRMA.org*, accessed August 3, 2016 http://www.phrma.org/cost.

30. David H. Howard, Peter B. Back, Ernst R. Berndt, and Rena M. Conti, "Pricing in the Market for Anticancer Drugs," *Journal of Economic Perspectives* 29, no. 1 (2015): 139–62.

31. Hagop Kantarjian, David Steensma, Judit Rius Sanjuan, Adam Elshaug, and Donald Light, "High Cancer Drug Prices in the United States: Reasons and Proposed Solutions," *Journal of Oncology Practice* 10, no. 4 (2014): 208–11.

32. Ibid.

33. PhRMA, "Counterfeit Drugs," *PhRMA.org*, accessed August 3, 2016 http://phrma.org/counterfeit-drugs.

34. Center for Responsive Politics, "Pharmaceutical Rsrch & Mfrs of America," *OpenSecrets.org*, accessed August 3, 2016 http://www.opensecrets.org/lobby/clientsum.php?id=D000000504&year=2016.

35. Ibid.

36. David H. Howard, Peter B. Back, Ernst R. Berndt, and Rena M. Conti, "Pricing in the Market for Anticancer Drugs," *Journal of Economic Perspectives* 29, no. 1 (2015): 139–62.

37. Cord Sturgeon, "Patients with Thyroid Cancer Are at Higher Risk of Bankruptcy than Patients with Other Types of Cancer, or Those Without Cancer," *Clinical Thyroidology* 25, no. 7 (2013): 150–51.

38. Scott D. Ramsey, Aasthaa Bansal, Catherine R. Fedorenko, David K. Blough, Karen A. Overstreet, Veena Shankaran, and Polly Newcomb, "Financial Insolvency as a Risk Factor for Early Mortality Among Patients With Cancer," *Journal of Clinical Oncology* 34 (2016): 1–7.

39. Ralph W. Moss, *The Cancer Industry* (Brooklyn: Equinox Press, 1996).

40. David H. Howard, Peter B. Back, Ernst R. Berndt, and Rena M. Conti, "Pricing in the Market for Anticancer Drugs," *Journal of Economic Perspectives* 29, no. 1 (2015): 139–62.

41. Peter A. Ubel, Amy P. Abernathy, and S. Yousef Zafar, "Full Disclosure-Out-of-Pocket Costs as Side Effects," *New England Journal of Medicine* 369, no. 16 (2013): 1484–86.

42. Hagop Kantarjian, David Steensma, Judit Rius Sanjuan, Adam Elshaug, and Donald Light, "High Cancer Drug Prices in the United States: Reasons and Proposed Solutions," *Journal of Oncology Practice* 10, no. 4 (2014): 208–11.

43. Ralph W. Moss, *The Cancer Industry* (Brooklyn: Equinox Press, 1996), 421.

44. Ibid.

Chapter Seven

1. Phil Brown and Edwin J. Mikkelsen, *No Safe Place: Toxic Waste, Leukemia, and Community Action* (Berkeley, CA: University of California Press, 1990), 43.

Index

Page numbers followed by "*t*" indicate a table. Page numbers followed by "*f*" indicate a figure.

About the Author

Wendy N. Whitman Cobb is assistant professor of political science at Cameron University, Lawton, Oklahoma. She received her PhD from the University of Florida and is the author of *Unbroken Government: Success and Failure in Policymaking*. Dr. Whitman Cobb's research has appeared in *Congress and the Presidency* and *Space Policy*.